July [illegible]/99

Happy Birthday Dad!

Love Your Daughters

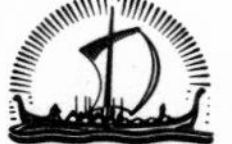

Toe Rubber Blues

mid-life thoughts on the prospects of aging

Tom Allen

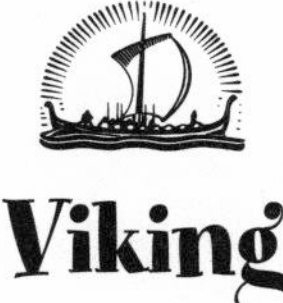

Viking

VIKING
Published by the Penguin Group
Penguin Books Canada Ltd, 10 Alcorn Avenue, Toronto, Ontario, Canada M4V 3B2
Penguin Books Ltd, 27 Wrights Lane, London W8 5TZ, England
Penguin Putnam Inc., 375 Hudson Street, New York, New York 10014, U.S.A.
Penguin Books Australia Ltd, Ringwood, Victoria, Australia
Penguin Books (NZ) Ltd, cnr Rosedale and Airborne Roads, Albany, Auckland 1310, New Zealand

Penguin Books Ltd, Registered Offices: Harmondsworth, Middlesex, England

First published 1999
1 3 5 7 9 10 8 6 4 2

Printed and bound in Canada on acid-free paper ∞

CANADIAN CATALOGUING IN PUBLICATION DATA

Allen, Tom, 1961–
Toe rubber blues: mid-life thoughts on the prospects of aging

ISBN 0-670-87897-9

1. Aging – Humour. I. Title.

PS8551.L55572T63 1998 C818'.5402 C98-930988-6
PR9199.3.A3965R82

Visit Penguin Canada's website at www.penguin.ca

To my parents

Contents

Acknowledgments

SPECIAL THANKS TO MY WIFE, children, sister, parents and in-laws, who have seen so much of what they say and do come back to haunt them.

Jeff Reilly, Nancy Watson, Cathy Perry, Carole Warren and Michelle Parise have all, over the years as my producers at the CBC, worked and put up with me. Many of the ideas that appear in one form or another in this book began in conversation and work with them. The same is true for Meg Masters, who is, in my mind, the only editor a radio host needs to know. Thanks also to Scott Sellers at Penguin, and to Cynthia Good for making everything, and almost anything, possible.

"Delivered From Evil," "Working the Room," "Still Too Young to Get Dressed," "Here We Go," "Ties" and "Toe Rubbers" all first appeared, for the most part, on the CBC Radio One program "Fresh Air," heard in Ontario and Quebec.

Thanks also to: Barbara Brown, Alan Foster, Rod Hinton, Janet Muse, the CBC Reference Library, Adrian Shuman, Dr. Charles Scriver for courage beyond the call of duty in attempting to teach a trombonist the basics of genetics, Ed Keall, Dr. Alexander Logan, Heather Barnes,

Josh Barnes, Terri Favro and Ron Edding for the kindness of good neighbours, John the suffering father, Tom Williams at Merrill Lynch (manager of the Fun, Fun, Fund), Bert Hall for taking the time, John Einarson (Kurt Lives!) and George Bubenik for explaining armpits.

Introduction

I am getting old.

But that's okay. My friend Will is, too.

Will's in good shape, but his eyes are showing some lines at the edges, and lately his hair has been greying slightly, too.

On the inside, however, Will is the same age he's always been. Inside, behind the grumbling muscles and the failing eyes, Will is, I figure, about six years old. This is by no means meant as an insult. He is in no way immature. Will pays his bills, maintains his marriage and is, by all accounts, a wonderful man to work with and for. But when an idea strikes Will, he plays with it all day. He carries it with him like a six-year-old would a pebble off the beach, pulling it in and out of his pocket until it is worn smooth. Then he looks for another one.

As far as I can tell, Will's pockets are so full of pebbles—from socio-political theories to fragments of show tunes—and they come and go at such a rate, that sometimes my only hope is to remember what I can about the identifying features of the one I'm most interested in and hang on through all the others until it turns up again.

Since getting to know him, I've begun to wonder if

everyone doesn't have an "inside age" that is there from the beginning. Think of Pierre Trudeau rolling down the window of his limousine to tell the press to *mange d'la merde*, marrying someone who turned out to be a lot keener on the Rolling Stones than on the Prime Minister and, when times got really tough, running off on a canoe trip and trying to grow a beard.

A spoiled sixteen-year-old comes to mind.

George Bush, on the other hand, spent his years in office acting like a skinny twelve-year-old student council president with lots of big friends, and Celine Dion has wanted to be forty-five since she turned fifteen.

None of this is to say that it is in any way bad to be forty-five on the inside—or twelve, or sixteen. It just has to be accounted for, which is far easier to drop as an idea into a book introduction than to actually do.

I've found that an awareness of clothes can help.

The way I figure it, clothes have an inside age too, regardless of current fashion. A grey flannel suit will always be right in the middle, about fifty, and a wide-lapelled, cream-coloured, three-piece suit, although it wants desperately to be legal age and get into the bar with its friends, will always be more comfortable at a junior high prom.

This isn't to say that a person must wear only the clothes that match their inside age. If that were so, Brian Mulroney would have spent the 1980s dressed in a jean jacket and a backwards baseball cap, with a toothpick between his teeth—a back-row, grade-seven thug trying to get in with the tall, white-haired guy in the red, white and blue tailcoat sitting at the desk to the south. No. Clothes can't alter character. But if they're well chosen, they can keep a person from slipping on a banana peel of self-deception and winding up with a nasty stain on their seat.

And since you're about to read an entire book about this sort of thing, or at least you might have thought you wanted to, I feel obliged to tell you that, although I have pioneered the theory of inside-age carbon dating, I really have no idea what my own inside age is, except that it feels most comfortable when I'm wearing my toe rubbers.

I think this is a good thing.

If this theory of aging is worth anything, it would stand to reason that when inner age and actual age coincide, things might end up being pretty good for a little while.

I'm thirty-seven, married, the father of two, and a morning show radio host.

It's too late for me to be the child genius, the teenage thug, the college football star, the young professional, and so far I don't feel like I am a mature, relaxed and comfortable father and husband.

What's left, then?

Well, how old *is* a man when he starts feeling good in his toe rubbers?

Right.

And you know what? I think that's okay. I don't mind not being young any more, and I'm not old, either. If this is mid-life, it's not so bad. At least from here I can honestly appreciate both ends of the journey. And, in keeping with the kind of rationalization that has helped humans stay mostly sane since the beginning of time, I have come up with an entire book outlining the reasons why that is okay. I will tell you why obsolete technologies like the slide rule and the turntable, and the people who used them, have intrinsic value that goes beyond usefulness. I will tell you why work isn't everything, and how, no matter what the RRSP commercials say, it *is* too late for you to save any money for your retirement. I will tell you why bald is *really* sexy, why "family planning" is an oxymoron, why time is irrelevant, where you should spend the winters of your senior years, what suite you will have in the exclusive downtown residences of the afterlife and how long it will be until you will be comfortable in your hat, your Friday wear, your ties or with no clothes on at all, depending on where you choose to spend your winters.

And, for the time being, until I become the quizzical, hirsute, eyebrow-cocking literary scamp in his twilight years who never answers a question with anything less puzzling than a parable, I will tell you all about my toe rubbers, just in case you want to get a pair, too.

Toe Rubber Blues

Dear Old Gear

My mom replaced the Moffat refrigerator last summer.

It was a big decision. Oh sure, it frosted up easily and groaned in the middle of the night, but who doesn't once they're thirty-nine? And besides, even though it was old, it was doing about as well as it had since I finished high school. I'm not sure what the formula is for converting fridge years to human years, but it can't be very stringent. That Moffat was young for one or two years, aging for another four and old for the next thirty-three, until it was executed for freezing the lettuce.

I've never met anyone who worked in the Moffat factory in the late 1950s, but I suspect one of their fridges lasting thirty-nine years wouldn't surprise them. There are probably more fridges left around from that time than workers. That's how they were built—to last. The fridges, I mean.

But a mere forty human years (or 1.025 Moffat refrigerator lifetimes) later, the appliance manufacturers have decided that dependability and longevity are no longer economically desirable. Maintenance has been deemed an unnecessary expense. You won't have to throw your current fridge away—it is programmed to experience feelings of inadequacy as soon as a younger model is issued, and it will leave on its own shortly after the warranty expires. You'll find your food neatly stacked on the counter the next morning, with the mouldy preserves thrown into the garbage, and a note on the floor, in a boxy hand, saying "I'm Sorry."

Being only slightly younger than my parents' recently discarded fridge, with an inside age that is probably slightly older, I'd like to hope this needn't be so. I think age is important in this kind of equipment—the stuff I like to call "gear." Dents and scrapes have stories to tell. They're a reminder of times gone by.

Besides, any gear that's any good needs character, and character takes time. Without time to age and mellow it a little, a machine is stuck with something very close to the personality it got from the human who made it. The CBC's in-house software program comes to mind. It's about five years old now (.128 in Moffat refrigerator lifetimes, 250,000,000,000 in computer software years). I don't think I've ever met its designer, but I feel reasonably confident I could identify him. At some office function one day, I'm sure, I'll ask someone a question only to have them stare blankly at me for several minutes and finally say "Hello" again and reintroduce themselves as if we'd never met. Bingo.

With that system still gainfully (and forcibly) employed, while the indestructible Moffats are put out to pasture, it is easy to lose hope. My only comfort is the knowledge that character, however outdated, doesn't simply evaporate. Somehow, that old Moffat, I feel sure, will find a way to be of use. If nothing else, it will have plenty of stories to share with its young and character-deprived neighbours in the junk yard. Or perhaps it might run a hotline for those depressive fridges who call out in the middle of the night, suddenly unsure of themselves, desperate and sweaty and wanting to know how to pick up a pen.

Sliding Home

My parents sold the family home, the one I'll never be able to afford, when I was nineteen. They moved to Toronto, to a condo that would have fit into our old basement, with a storage locker in the basement that would have fit into our old bathroom.

A lot of my stuff had to go.

I wasn't ready to part with much of it and have since blanked from memory most of the garage sale that followed. I do remember Tommy Webster wanting my junior-sized baseball bat, the one he claimed I'd stolen years before, which I hadn't. I'd bought it at Wilson's Sporting Goods with my dad. It cost four dollars then, but I offered it to Tommy that day at the garage sale for fifty. Dollars. It went to Mom and Dad's new place.

So did my Town of Mount Royal Pee Wee Jets 1974 Provincial Champs football jacket, which is not as impressive as it sounds. My team won the championship for the eight-man league. There aren't many leagues that play eight-man football. I suspect those that do are created for teams like ours, which had tried the standard twelve-man league the previous year and had been pasted by each and every opponent. Our season in the twelve-man league culminated in a campaign against the mighty North Shore squad, in which they danced around us, singing songs, *during the game*, while we attempted a screen pass. We gained no yards at all and lost eighty-eight to nothing.

Then we switched leagues, and won. I got a jacket. It kept the bat company on the trip to my parents' new place. And so did my slide rule.

I might have tried to sell the slide rule in the garage sale, perhaps to Tommy Webster, I'm not sure. But if I did, I'm glad I failed. Because now, from its position as museum piece in my sock drawer, that slide rule, I can finally appreciate, is a beautiful thing. It's a British Thornton ten-inch, with full logarithmic and trigonometrical scales and two-sided cursor bar for maximum efficiency. It has the feel of the steering wheel on a fine sports car. When you pick it up, your hands know they're holding something worthwhile. The surface is buffed smooth. The slide glides easily back and forth. And the real thrill is, it works! It's just a bunch of numbers on a stick, but you move this here, you move that there, and *bam!* Math!

Incredible.

The slide rule did that for people for about three hundred and forty years, starting with William Oughtred. He invented it in 1630. He was an Episcopal minister, and he was English, which, to the chaps at British Thornton, was a good thing. Here's the back page of their instruction manual:

MAJOR HISTORICAL DEVELOPMENTS
IN THE HISTORY OF THE SLIDE RULE

*1614 Invention of logarithms by John Napier, Baron of Merchiston, Scotland

*1617 Development of logarithms "to base 10" by Henry Briggs, Professor of Mathematics, Oxford University

*1620 Interpretation of logarithmic scale form by Edmund Gunter, Professor of Astronomy, London

*1630 Invention of slide rule by the Reverend William Oughtred, London

*1657 Development of the moving slide/fixed stock principle by Seth Partridge, Surveyor and Mathematician

*1775 Development of the slide rule cursor by John Robertson of the Royal Academy

1815 Invention of the log log scale principle by P.M. Roget of France

*1900 Re-introduction of log log scales by Professor Perry, Royal College of Science, London

*1933 Differential trigonometrical and log log scales invented by Hubert Boardman, Radcliffe, Lancashire

---

* denotes British development

Whew! Good thing old Professor Perry had the foresight to "re-introduce" the log log scale principle eighty-five years after P.M. Roget invented it. Then again, it's not as if history would have been foolish enough to give Roget any real credit, anyway. Professor Perry was from the Royal College of Science, for God's sake, and any fool can see that Roget, the poor sod, was only "of France."

Not so William Oughtred. His developments were as British as they come. Rather than coming from London, as the Thorntonites would have it, he was born in Eton, educated there and at Cambridge, and ended up the rector of Albury, in Surrey, a not-so-shabby church appointment. His passion, however, was math. He invented all kinds of theories and symbols, including the "x" we use for multiplication and the "::" for proportion. He was a committed tutor, and, although he consistently refused to be paid for his teaching, his list of students included many noted mathematicians, as well as the architect Christopher Wren.

William Oughtred lived to be ninety-six years old. You'd probably need more than a slide rule to figure out how he did that. Ninety-six wasn't exactly the average life expectancy in the 1600s. It makes you wonder if some historian along the line screwed up while calculating the dates using a slide rule. It sure is easy to do. You get flinging that slide around and digits come and go like limousines at a bank presidents' lunch.

You have to hand it to Oughtred for one thing, though: he was thinking long-term. The slide rule is the perfect tool for the late-twentieth century. It doesn't care whether that's 9.6 at the bottom of the column or 96,000,000,000. The zeroes are up to you, whether you're balancing a federal budget or financing a resort development.

I don't want to come off as holier, arithmetically speaking, than thou. I don't have a slide rule because I enjoy the slower pace of manual/logarithmic calculation, or because I want to read the sines along the way. I haven't used the thing in twenty-one years, except for occasionally reminding myself how it works by figuring something I already know ("10/2 = 50? Wait a minute . . ."). My British Thornton might be beautiful, but it's also cruel and unforgiving, and I bought it only because I had to, weeks before my grade ten mid-term exams.

Canadians are the kind of people who generally believe that you can't get anywhere without back-breaking, unfulfilling work. But, just to be sure no one misses out, they now and then favour policies like the one our school board adopted in 1977. Hand-held calculators had existed for a few years, but they weren't allowed in exams, because, well, because a slide rule was a lot harder to use, thus teaching the young Canadian the value of racking one's brains and still screwing up.

It's not as if Montreal's anglophone community needed to make the future any bleaker for its young people. In fact, those mid-terms came right after the first electoral victory of the separatist Parti Québécois. It makes you wonder whether they were upset over that Roget and Perry stuff in the instruction manual. Especially considering that, one year later, the school board recommended that we switch from British Thornton to Texas Instruments.[1] That's right, just one year later, calculators were suddenly acceptable, making the young Canadian feel he might have been better off to have failed the exam and taken it again the easy way.

I'd have needed to take a year off to work before I could afford my own hand-held calculator, though. I still remember the first time I saw one. It was on the back page of the Eaton's catalogue: the Rapidman 800. It would add, subtract, divide and multiply. It fit in your pocket, and it cost one hundred dollars.

---

[1] Paving the way for classification of mathematical discoveries with the priority placed on those that might be considered "Texan Developments."

A hundred bucks! You could fly to Europe in those days for a hundred bucks! And even if it rained, you'd end up with more memories than the Rapidman 800. It had no memory at all.

A lot of people bought them anyway. In the spring after that grade ten mid-term I went on a work-study program in the architecture division at Canadian National Railways. My responsibilities included wearing a suit, catching the train and being first in line at the doughnut trolley in the lobby at ten o'clock. In exchange I was allowed to spend two weeks in the company of some twenty master architects, and watch as they put their burning creativity to work on a continuing series of freight sheds, pedestrian overpasses and parking lots. It was grim. Most of the people working there were young men, already nestled into the bowels of bureaucracy with no prospect of significant movement ahead. They compensated with banter, with cynicism, with cigarettes, and with gear.

Of course, what passed for gear in those days would seem quaintly futile today. The drafting tables were right out of a Dickensian accountant's office. Each one had a mechanical T-square that was wired like the mast of a schooner and weighed about as much. And the top of the table was equipped, for convenience, with a tilt adjustment that invariably dumped steaming coffee into the lap of the unfortunate worker, and, shortly thereafter, pulverized the knees.

The other now-archaic tool used throughout the office was the pencil. Most guys had dozens on the go, of various weights, each one needing almost constant sharpening. This took two steps, two hands and two different sharpeners. The first looked like a classroom model gone bad, all cranks, rods and pinchers. It ground away only the wood, leaving a great limb of exposed lead about half an inch long. The second sharpener was shaped in the style of an elfin wood stove with a circular sanding track inside. The pencil, if the exposed lead had not yet been broken, was dropped gingerly into the chimney and turned around the track for long enough to calcify the joints of the user. At this point, the pencil had been shortened to the length of a thumb, the point made lethally sharp, and work could resume, for about ten minutes, until the pencil broke again.

You can see how the blazing technology of the mighty Rapidman 800, memory or not, shone by comparison. Everybody in the office had one, except for Josef and Taddeus and me.

Josef and Taddeus were from Poland. They'd come to Canada in the early 1950s and were, by then, just a few years from retirement. They were by far the oldest men in the office, and by far the least burdened with gear. Unlike the rest of us, they cast their schooner-sized T-squares out to sea and drew freehand. They used onionskin paper held in place with pins. They sharpened with a penknife, the same one they used to carve apples at lunch. And when they calculated something, they used a slide rule. They shared a pocket-sized model between them, snatched back and forth between the desks, the slide darting in and out like the needles in a knitting machine.

One morning there was a crash down the hall and some screaming. Somebody's Rapidman 800 had drowned in a coffee spill and cost the owner another trip to Europe. Josef smiled. "My calculator loves coffee," he said, and he sloshed the slide rule around in his mug, like a stir stick. "Lubricates the mechanism."

They laughed at my slide rule for being so spotless. It even smelled new. It still does, a little bit. And, as impressive as it is to find something both brand new and two decades old, I find it a little bit sad. My British Thornton, for all the political strife it witnessed in its one season of use, never had the chance to age. I'm sure it would have been much happier stirring Josef's coffee, but that wasn't to be. It was obsolete before I finished high school, and it's lived in dresser drawers and boxes ever since, entombed alongside its fellow garage sale survivors: a thirty-year-old allegedly stolen junior-sized baseball bat and a championship football jacket, won by bureaucratic lobbying and compromise. They lie there in the dark, the three of them, whispering of their pasts, calculating their own street value as antiques and wondering where to put the decimal.

Oh, the Pedalo!

As the years go by, I would like to be perceived as aging gracefully. I'd like to *actually* age gracefully, too, but first things first. Actual gracefulness requires integrity, wisdom and inner peace, which are all very well, but who's going to know you've got them when you can hardly move because your knees are wooden, your back is throbbing, and your feet feel like salad forks? There are a lot of old people out there these days. As integrated, wise and internally peaceful as they may be, if they bellow and moan and curse like longshoremen with every lurching step on the way to the gracefulness seminar, chances are, by the time they reach the registration table, their pass to the plenary session will have mysteriously disappeared.

Among aging humans, graceful movement is the first thing to go.

But there are ways to get around the problem of getting around. I once knew an orchestra conductor who aged beautifully. I had no idea how old he was, except that he wasn't young. When I first met him he had long, flowing white hair, hawk eyebrows, talon hands, bony joints, piercing eyes and the air of someone you were lucky to have met while he was still alive. The next time we met, fifteen years later, he looked exactly the same. I'm sure he still does.

He was a brilliant extemporaneous speaker who seemed absolutely unafraid of saying anything to anyone. In Halifax he gave an already starched and terrified audience a series of pre-concert talks on syphilis and the great composers. I once heard him lecture an orchestra of teenagers on the composer Anton Bruckner, the need to suffer and masturbation. (". . . And, in those days," he explained, "masturbation was not the exalted thing it is today, it was a very grave sin! I think, now, we may have gone too far in the other direction. *[wistfully]* Perhaps, one day, masturbation will find its place in society.") And in Toronto's Roy Thomson Hall, to a packed house, with the assembled musicians waiting on stage, he gave a ten-minute introduction to the *Battle Symphony* ("Wellington's Victory") by Beethoven, which concluded with the line: "And, ladies and gentlemen, let me say to you, what you are about to hear is not good music." Then we heard it. He was right.

Now, this man didn't have much in the way of gear. He didn't even conduct with a baton. But when he had to travel, he rode a bicycle.

His was the fold-up kind, with tiny wheels and a sky-high seat that made it look like an escaped exercycle. It looked to be about as old as he was. But when he went by, with white hair and black shorts, probably humming a tune by Bruckner (and thinking, well, who knows?), he was a graceful sight. People would stop on the sidewalk and look, and smile, and when they came across his Ichabod bike, they gave it room. He never locked it, that I saw, and as far as I know it was never stolen. In fact, to this day, if it were put up for sale in a city where he had been conductor—along with, say, a copy of *Crime and Punishment* and a couple of self-help manuals—I'm sure it would fetch a fine dollar.

To assume that this particular bicycle would lend gracefulness to anyone but its original owner, however, would be a bit of a leap.[1]

As an alternative, most aging North Americans in search of graceful motion opt for one of the mainstays of this century's manufacturing-based economy. That might sound honourable. It is not. Cars are singularly graceless. The exertion of your foot on the gas pedal is the exertion of the oil-supplying nations on your government, of the government on your tax bill, of your tax bill on your gas bill, of your gas bill on your exhaust levels, of your exhaust levels on the ozone layer, of the ozone layer on your conscience, of your conscience on your attention span, of your attention span on the fellow in your blind spot, of the fellow in your blind spot on your rear fender, of your rear fender on the body shop, of the body shop back onto your bills, conscience, attention span and already toxic stress levels, resulting in wooden knees, a throbbing back and feet that feel like salad forks.

And, if you're over forty, a flashy new sports car is not a sign of success and arrival, or even a practical means of conveyance. It is a sign of:

1. Fear of age. Thus transported, you may think you're going to purr into the driveway of maturity, but you are deceived. You get in that foolish machine and put on those sunglasses and there is a mid-life crisis waiting for

---

[1] You would probably have to lecture on Bruckner, or something, as well, and not be arrested for it.

you just beyond the curb. Your ridiculous new car is going to break down before you leave the garage and you won't be able to fix it because it's built of modular components that are kept in vaults overseas, and if you drive it downtown on a sunny day you'll have people muttering about the size of your drive shaft.

But, if you stay with your old car, it is a sure sign of:

2. Fear of freedom. Come on, you can't just sit around waiting for life to tell you what to do! Look at you—eating tea and toast and forgetting your children's names while you drool on your bedclothes and wait for the bridge club to come over so you can eat commercially made Nanaimo bars dripping with modified oils and artificial sweeteners that turned healthy and vigorous laboratory rats into bitter, old, urine-stained geezers years ago. You are sucking the life out of your loved ones, and maybe you've been masquerading as a caring person all these years, but we can all see now that you're just a selfish old windbag.

So, if you ditch your old car, to avoid number 2, you'll invariably need a new one, and then you're back to number 1. And if you manage to hang on to the slippery slope of new-car-assisted moral collapse, and age gracefully along with that evil, new machine, you'll probably have to throw *it* out eventually, anyway, and then you're right back where you started.

When it comes to aging and transportation, a car will bring you grief and grief alone, and gracefulness will have long since driven off the lot.

The other option, as I see it, is to get a boat. Boats are naturally high in apparent gracefulness. They don't walk or step or even roll to get around, they simply float. And even when that fails, they don't jerk or screech or crash into the guardrail in a hail of sparks and searing steel; they tip, like a teacup.

Of course, there are horrifically graceless boats. One does have to exercise a certain amount of judgment when making one's choice. Just as an expensive sports car will bring its driver invariably to moral degradation, so will a rumbling, water-borne monster send any hope of gracefulness running back to the cottage for earplugs. No. Spending a lot of money and making a lot of noise will not solve the problem. In fact, with boats, the opposite is often true. The modest canoe is industrious and unassuming, the rowing scull stoic and efficient, and, among boats, there are few, in my opinion, that rival the frugality, the inner peace and, indeed, the wisdom, integrity and gracefulness of the pedal boat.

My parents have one at their home in rural Quebec, where a pedal boat is called a "pedalo," from "*pied à l'eau*," or "foot in the water," which can happen. The classic pedalo is built like a slow-motion catamaran. There are two pontoons held together with a wooden frame, a paddle wheel between and a set of pedals on each side. There is deck space and a pair of wooden seats.

Our family friend Florian gave us the pedalo twenty-five years ago, for nothing, after we promised to fix it up. If we wanted to use it, there wasn't a whole lot of choice. It had been sitting in the grass behind his house for eight years. Or about eight years. That was all he was willing to admit to at the time. That and the fact that his father had found it abandoned in the bulrushes in a swamp years before that.

The original frame was as rotten as a pie crust left in the rain. But the pontoons, the ones that had actually been sitting in the grass and snow and, before that, for an undisclosed amount of time, possibly longer than eight years, in the swamp, were in amazingly good shape. They were made of a marine-grade plywood that was so strong and waterproof the company that made it had cash problems. What kind of business can you build when your customers only come back every nine years? It went under.

But the pontoons didn't. Not right away, anyway. With the help, every spring, of ten or twelve pounds of fibreglass to seal up the edges, and more than a few coats of paint, they lasted six more years. By then, they weighed so much that the pedalo floated comfortably at about two and a half feet below the surface, making it really a "*tout à l'eau*," and causing problems in shallow bays.

So, we went to see Henri Berthiome. Henri was the local boat-builder, and his workshop was a place of wonder. There were rowboats stacked in the corners, the gassy smell of resin hanging low over the worktables and about two hundred canoe paddles hanging from the rafters.

The paddles were of his own design, with a slight angle where the blade met the shaft, and the rowboats were the local cash crop in the boat-building trade: a wide, flat design called a chaloupe. A Berthiome chaloupe was indestructible, and was as comfortable at the fishing hole, casting for trout, as it was taking the family in to Chez Walter for dinner. For a pair of pontoons, Henri Berthiome was eminently qualified. He made us a pair that could have crossed the Atlantic.

Unfortunately, those pontoons might have been better

off if they had. That first winter, Dad stored them under the cottage, where a porcupine found them and decided they suited his purposes, too.

Porcupines are rodents, believe it or not, and although I guess I'd rather have one under the cottage eating a potentially graceful watercraft than, say, scurrying around the kitchen cabinets with the other rodents, the whole thing is a little hard to understand. Sure, rodents need to chew things or their teeth get too long. But still—a boat?

When I was growing up in Montreal there was a guy who used to show up as entertainment at the Auto Show. He was an average-looking fellow who called himself "Monsieur Mangetout"—"Mr. Eat Everything." And he did. He ate little things like drinking glasses and drywall screws as teasers at the trade shows, but his real passion were the long-term projects he had on the slow burner. As of 1996, he had eaten ten bicycles, seven television sets, six chandeliers, a shopping cart, a coffin (including the handles) and, the height of his digestive achievement, a plane. It was a two-passenger Cessna. He ate it, and the rest, at a rate of one kilogram per day, enjoying servings of one or two bolts at a time.

"Monsieur Mangetout" didn't crawl under cabins in the black of night to do his chewing—he was diurnal, for one thing, but he was proud of himself, too. It was his career. He even got into the *Guinness Book of Records*. So, I don't know what that porcupine's problem was. I'd pay good money to see a porcupine eat a boat. As long as it wasn't mine.

The naturalists I spoke to said it might have been the glue in the plywood the porcupine was after, but it might have been the salt on the corners from M. Berthiome's hands, too. There are lots of stories of wanton gustatorial destruction committed by porcupines. One person found a six-inch hole in the middle of a brand new porch where a drop of barbecue sauce had been spilled. Another lost the better part of a plywood toilet seat from the outhouse. The idea of a porcupine in the outhouse is uncomfortable enough, thank you very much, without bringing up the idea of razor-sharp teeth.

Anyway, the point, so to speak, of all this is that our pedalo never had the pleasure of seeing the new, lightweight pontoons added to its arsenal of grace-inducing features. By the time we floated it again that spring, the pontoons needed another metric tonne or so of fibreglass to keep them together.

Even with a little extra weight, though, a pedalo is a wonderful boat. It's completely impractical for work of any kind—slow to start, slow to stop and, most wonderfully, slow to go. The best you might accomplish is a gentle pace that can hardly fail to soothe the anxious mind. And the other, most gracious feature of pedalo travel is that it encourages conversation. In fact, to put it less than gracefully, it forces it. There is no way to toss off a quick "Hi" to the folks on shore if you're in a pedalo. Once you start talking, there is no way to escape in a hurry. You're in for the long haul, whether you like it or not. Conversational etiquette is simply the only reasonable course.

Pedal boats first turned up in eighteenth-century Europe. They were mostly hand-powered, though, and it doesn't sound as though they could honestly have been called pleasure craft. But when Queen Victoria's eldest son, Edward, the Prince of Wales, got hold of one, things began to change. Edward, it seems, wasn't all that reliable, or pleasant, had trouble with anything resembling prolonged mental exertion and really wasn't very practical for work of any kind, himself—but he was a demon with a pedal boat.

He had his own fleet. He called them Water-Velocipedes, and you can bet the only swamp they ever encountered was a social one. The Water-Velocipede was the patented invention of Searle & Sons, the Royal Boat Builders, and it boasted beautiful woodwork, unparalleled comfort and distinctive styling. Edward had two-seaters, four-seaters, one with a special spot for the Royal Dog and a solo model, which he's reported to have used at regular intervals to escape (slowly) both the neighbours and the rigours of Royal Life.

After his time, since most people couldn't afford the services of the Royal Boat Builders, some pretty interesting contraptions turned up. In 1910 a Mr. Rowell of Cambridgeshire put a bicycle frame on pontoons and called it a watercycle. He was photographed, looking quite dapper in a grey wool suit, while plying the River Ouse. And in Toronto, around the same time, there were ferryboats pedalled by horses. The pilot put one horse over each paddle-wheel and had the beast walk, as if on a treadmill. It was, we can be relatively sure, Toronto's first two-horsepower engine.

The last forty years, however, have been cruel to the pedalo. With the invention of moulded plastic, the days of the adventurous and graceful-if-eccentric pedalo were numbered. Like everything else, all pedal boats started to look the same, especially while being swamped by a Sea-Doo (or Personal Water Craft). To our family, one of those production-line, rectangular, modified-yogurt-container pedalos (*pedaleaux?*) with a tinny paddle and orange, moulded plastic seats was almost unthinkable. But by late 1996, it appeared we had no choice. Our second (I think) generation of plywood pontoons had expired. Sadly, by then, Henri Berthiome had too. We were stuck.

Then something happened that makes me wonder about true gracefulness, integrity, wisdom, the finding of things in the bulrushes and even inner peace. My parents' neighbour moved away and abandoned his pedalo, strangely enough, in the bulrushes behind his house. The frame was useless and the paddle was bent, but the pontoons—great, huge, aluminum monsters—were perfect. It was like changing tires. True, the people that have moved in now do have Sea-Doos, and a knack for blasting around the bay like horseflies over rot, ruining the shoreline with their wakes and sucking any incidental gracefulness (to say nothing of inner peace) out of a Saturday afternoon in almost no time at all, but the Lord has always worked in mysterious waves.

Now, the pedalo appears to be back in the swim. For one thing, in 1997 the pedalo's natural enemy, Bombardier's cursed Personal Water Craft, was finally dropped out of production. Between saturating the market (and the market's neighbours) and slinging muck of one kind or another all over that company's once-credible name, the silly Sea-Doo obviously sank itself. And, not long before that, the modest pedalo began to make waves of its own. One summer evening in southern Italy, three pirates raided a British yacht, bound and gagged the passengers and made off with £50,000! Their vehicle? That's right. A few months after that, two Englishmen actually *did* pedal across the Atlantic. And, just when I thought eccentricity had lumbered away from pedal boats altogether, I discovered the International Human Powered Vehicle Association. They sponsor speed trials. The record is over 20 mph, and the range of eccentric vessels is staggering. There's a human-powered submarine in the works, and one industrious fellow in Finland has come up with a hydrofoil that is powered by jumping. The driver grips a set of bicycle-like handles, but instead of turning pedals to generate speed, he bounces up and down, standing on a sprung metal base that, if there is enough bouncing, rides just above the water's surface. The inventor calls it the Trampofoil. He has a web site, too. You can see little video clips of him jumping across a frigid Finnish canal. Which, to be honest, is not exactly what most people would call a graceful sight, but it does look like fun.

And that, I guess, ends up being part of the pursuit of gracefulness, too. Maybe it's just my work-ethic upbringing, but it seems to me that if any of us is actually going to make the transition from apparent to real gracefulness, it's probably going to happen while we're busy doing something else. Whether that means you're better off jumping across canals, riding a tall bike and whistling Bruckner, shopping for sports cars and adjusting your pants, *fwup-fwupping* around the bay, talking nicely or eating a bus, well, I don't know. But, whichever it is, I can't see any point in rushing. From what I've heard, getting there is half the fun.

For Every Season There Was a Turntable

I came across an old friend one evening last summer. It was a Sansui stereo amplifier, exactly like the one I bought with my paper route money twenty-four years ago. I instantly thought of our rec room in Montreal, of Jimi Hendrix, of wooden panelling, faux fireplaces and the smell from the cold room under the stairs. It was funny, because this Sansui came with its own distinctive smell, too. It was in my neighbour's garbage. He'd exiled it there after his daughter moved out and left it behind.

I wanted to take it home and plug it in, to see if it worked, but I couldn't. *My* daughter wouldn't hear of it. She wanted to look for the cricket.

The cricket turns up every August in our back yard. Every August my daughter wants me, even though it's long past her bedtime, and I've already given her a snack and a drink in the hope that she'll let me work on this book for more than a few minutes at a time so I won't have to keep writing run-on sentences, to take her outside to try to find him.

We never have.

This pattern disturbs me.

Not the fact that we haven't found him. It's almost

impossible, as you might know, to find a cricket in the dark. First of all, being well adapted to nocturnal activity, they are as black as tar. At least, the one in my back yard is. I think. After two straight summers of him chirping back there, I looked him up. There are about 2,400 different species of cricket, and without ever having seen him, it's hard to be certain which he is. But given our back yard's location within the generally accepted cricket habitat and the specifics of his song, I think he's a Field Cricket (genus *Gryllus*).

They're pretty cool, field crickets. I'd never noticed until I looked them up, but they have three different songs: one for attracting mates, one for mating and one for scaring off competing crickets. You can also tell how hot it is by how fast they are chirping.[1] And, they have highly sensitive sensors in their legs that tell them that what they've attracted isn't another cricket but, say, a bat, or some other beast keen on crickets for reasons other than the procreation of the species.

Our intent was never so malicious. We just liked seeing how close we could get before he stopped chirping.

We never got very close.

That's because our cricket is a good cricket. To him,[2] an approaching human would be something like what a monster with legs the size of office buildings would be to us.

---

[1] The formula for determining the temperature in Fahrenheit, I'm told, is to count the number of chirps over a period of fifteen seconds, and add 32. Good luck. If it's any warmer than 60 degrees, there are far too many chirps to count with any accuracy. If it's below 60 degrees, it's too cool to be out in the back yard in your pajamas, anyway. Buy a thermometer.

[2] It is "him," by the way. In field crickets, it's the guys that do all the chirping.

Let's imagine two humans on a date. Buster is carrying high hopes that he and Betty will attempt to create further human life before the night is through (although, likely, he's not particularly concerned with the long-term consequences of that attempt). We don't know Betty's opinion of Buster at the beginning of the evening, but once he shows indifference and boredom at the sight of a monster with legs the size of First Canadian Place, we can be relatively sure that Betty's interest in genetic co-production with Buster has waned.

So, unlike Buster, our cricket is a good and successful male of his species. In fact, I have learned since starting this piece[3] that "our cricket" is, in fact, not a single insect but a lineage. Crickets live for only six to eight weeks. That we have heard him (i.e., him and his sons) for two successive Augusts now, in the same location, is proof positive that he and, with each generation, at least one of his sons shut up the chirpers before the bats and the multistorey office buildings got them, wooed their dates sufficiently and got the job done.

None of that is what disturbs me. My worry is the extent to which the cricket calls interest my daughter. At the time of writing she is only three years old, and is clearly an easy mark when it comes to mating calls. An insect lineage or two in the back yard, fine. Hell, I wouldn't mind an entomology conference back there. But what's going to happen in twelve or thirteen years? I'll tell you what's going to happen: boys. Very loud boys with very loud sound systems in very loud cars, followed by headaches.

---

[3] Several moderately cool August nights ago.

What kind of noise it will be that brings on those headaches is much harder to predict.

I work with a friend who is the father of a teenage son. When his son turned thirteen, the boy became sullen, removed, antisocial, and he acquired an appetite such that, as my friend delicately put it, "All I saw when I came home was his bum sticking out of the fridge." All very normal. But this teenage son's taste in music, for almost an entire year, remained remarkably inert, non-threatening and even, at times, pleasant.

"I remember thinking," my friend told me, "maybe this wasn't going to be as bad as I thought." That's when the boy made his move. He'd been lying low all along, looking for a soft spot. You see, his father, my friend, is very open-minded about music, willing to listen to absolutely anything new and different. It took his son a good, long time to find what he was looking for. But once he did, their home became the headwaters for a raging torrent of musical stupidity—the boy took a liking to 1970s disco music.

"I'd come home from a long day and be reminded of myself in platform, two-tone shoes and wide-leg corduroy pants, doing 'The Bump' to 'A Fifth of Beethoven,'" the father told me. "It almost killed me."

But that was not, I believe, the boy's primary goal—an attractive by-product, perhaps. Playing what was arguably the worst popular music of the century at deafening volumes all hours of the day and night was, I'm convinced, primarily intended to find that teenage boy a mate.

I can't claim to be an expert in the area of human courtship rituals. Sometimes I think I'm lucky to have procreated at all. (Most male humans feel this way, or at least, as Buster would have, count themselves lucky to have tried.) But from the distance of a few years, it's all beginning to seem rather obvious to me.

Let's go back to our cricket.

Even if a male cricket is dimwitted, slow and, let's say, unusually fine-tasting to bats, if his chirp is good and loud he's a good investment for the average female. All he, or his offspring, has to do is survive a few days, find a mate and do the deed. A genius of the genus might have mastered calculus, or be on the verge of being able to communicate with those walking office buildings, but if he isn't loud enough to get a date, he's just chirping in the wind.[4]

It is a long way, I'll grant you, in evolutionary terms, from crickets to humans, and, aside from this noise-making thing, we don't seem to have a whole lot else in common. I'm not pushing any genetic link. Nevertheless, I think perhaps we humans haven't evolved as far from the

[4] Along the same lines, I spent a July in West Virginia years ago. That summer, a cicada-like beetle called "The Seventeen-Year Locust" came of age, and the place was covered in giant, buzzing bugs. I gather this happens only once every seventeen years, hence the name. Anyway, these locusts, as you can imagine, after having spent seventeen lonely years as underground grubs, were mighty keen on meeting the opposite sex, and they weren't about to sit waiting by the phone. The noise was deafening. It became clear, however, that the female was not so picky about what her mate looked like, or, for that matter, whether he was even remotely locust-like at all, as long as he was loud. They gleefully attached themselves by the dozens onto lawnmowers, leaf-blowers, air conditioners, jackhammers and just about anything else that roared with enough gusto to get their attention. Such lack of judgment would seem to bode ill for a species, but, apparently, the seventeen-year locust is doing just fine. They're due out again in the summer of 2000. West Virginia is nice in the summer. Why not head down yourself? Just bring some earplugs, and, if you're driving, check your muffler.

loudest-guy-gets-the-girl mentality as we'd like to think. At least the males haven't. We are still quite keen on noise. From the onset of puberty until he begins to roar not because he wants to mate but because he has thrown out his back, about all the average male wants to do is make noise . . . and mate. But, since he is never mating quite enough for his own liking, he has even more time for noise, and for discovering the many wonderful ways there are to make it.

A musical instrument is always high on the list of options, and, conveniently, for the purposes of the average male, actual musicianship is rarely deemed a necessity. Volume, however, is key, and if a phallic shape can be thrust into the mix—an electric guitar held at pelvis level, for example—so much the better.

The trombone, my own choice at the age of thirteen, is both tremendously phallic and tremendously loud. But it didn't get me very far. It might have attracted countless teenage beauties, I don't know. I was too busy playing as loud as I could to take any notice. Besides, getting their attention is one thing, but the next level of intimacy—be it conversation or any other oral activity—is difficult at best when you have a twelve-foot brass pipe attached to your mouth.

That is why most boys eschew the trombone, and even the electric guitar, for the most reliable source of deafening mating calls since 1877: the sound system.

Okay, maybe it wasn't quite enough to lure a potential mate into "the bachelor pad" in 1877. Come to think of it, it didn't do that much for me in 1977, either. But this isn't about success. It's about trying.

In 1877, Thomas Edison came up with his marvellous

Talking Machine. This little wonder would record and instantly replay the sound of the human voice to the amazement of everyone present, guys and gals alike. Edison, being beyond such things, didn't immediately recognize the salivating teenage boy as the major market for his invention. He hoped his machine would be used as a tool for dictation.

Within five years, however, a Talking Machine was in the hands of one Gianni Eduardo Bettini. Bettini lived in London, and, recognizing the potential for vast sales to people with romance on their minds, he went right to the source of the highest and loudest romance of the time: the Royal Opera at Covent Garden.

That was in 1881. He recorded singers, many of whom were women, and then, (presumably) in the privacy of their dressing rooms, treated them to the sound of their own lovely voices. Once Gianni had recovered from the exhausting trysts that (presumably) followed, he went home, took a bath, got dressed and waited for his next appointment.

Because the Edison Talking Machine recorded onto cylinders made of wax, each recording could be replayed only a few times before it wore out. So, if Mathilda or Nellie or Gertrude gave in to the temptation to hear her lovely voice more than a few times that night, she'd have to invite Gianni back to the next show to do it all again. And if you've ever known any opera singers of either gender, you know the only thing they enjoy more than trysts in the dressing room is the sound of their own voices.

Poor Gianni.

Of course, in 1881 we were still years from the fully functional bachelor pad with stackable easy-listening LPS and hideaway bed. But in terms of the evolution of the species, one important distinction had already taken hold. Bettini's recordings of the lovely operatic voices worked fine for his purposes. The vanity of his singers easily made up for a certain lack of clarity in the recorded sound. But as far as the mass market was concerned, Edison cylinders, and also the Emile Berliner flat disc system that followed it in 1894, had an important technological drawback: they worked well only with excessively loud music. Sweet violins and tender keyboard reflections just weren't heard. The earliest recording stars were brass bands, military bands, bombastic operatic orchestras and, by 1904, people like Enrico Caruso, who could yell high notes mostly in tune. Just like the industrious crickets of that era and ours, success in the recording industry, and, by extension, in the bachelor pad, required one qualification above all others: it was survival of the loudest.

Since then, of course, any problem with recording soft and subtle sounds has long been overcome. With every generation of sound technology innovation, the audiophile has come closer to transforming his living room or car into something very close to an actual concert hall. No matter. Somewhere back there, between Bettini and Buster, the damage was done.

I suppose it's possible that one day the guys I see hanging around the high school parking lot with the doors on their parents' car wide open will be marvelling over the extraordinary clarinet *pianissimo* in the opening of Tchaikovsky's *Romeo and Juliet*, but I'm not holding my breath. I don't think I have to tell you what I *do* hear. If you live anywhere within four miles of a high school parking lot, I'm sure you already know. And perhaps, like me, you worry about the structural security of your home when an industrious male student drives by in the middle of the night, woofers and tweeters all hooting for hooters.

The strange thing for me about all this tempest of testosterone is that I'm not sure it actually works. There might be a great number of young women that are helplessly drawn to men emitting big, deep, pulsating noises, but I haven't seen very many of them, and I've met even fewer. In fact, aside from the occasional blowhard who gets the nod, it's the Brad Pitts, Paul Newmans, Chet Bakers and even Marlon Brandos of this world who, more often than not, whisper a word or two per hour and have women wilting like daisies in a downpour.

All of which leaves me wondering where the genetic noise marker comes from in the first place. Maybe, way back when our DNA was only as powerful as a Sansui amplifier, yelling or whacking or banging was as important to genetic survival as a rock and a sharp stick. Maybe it's a leadership-of-the-herd thing, and it has more to do with impressing the other males than the females. Maybe we are all descendants of Jerry Lewis. Or maybe we males just haven't quite taken the latest evolutionary step.

Developmental experts have long held that girls mature faster than boys; maybe they have evolved faster, too. Maybe, if the Pitt, Brando & Co. quiet types father enough children, there will be enough of their whispering boys, with enough girls wilting around them, to actually get the attention of the seventeen-year-old boy-locusts and get them to turn the volume down a little.

It will be ten years before my daughter officially becomes a teenager. Ten years isn't very long in evolutionary terms, I know, but I'm hoping. Between global warming and El Niño and toxic waste and the turn of the millennium, I'm hoping for some bizarre mutation so that in August of 2008, in the evening, with my daughter waiting for *me* to go to sleep, I will stroll out into my back yard and, instead of feeling the earth tremble with the noise of passing sound systems, I will hear our cricket.

Perhaps I will be quiet enough, myself, by then, to get close enough to say hello. We will talk in whispers, he and I, and tell stories of the old days, before 1877, when life was peaceful, office buildings were shorter and bats were slower, and our ancestors enjoyed music, and love, and each other's company, in blessed, blessed quiet.

Delivered From Evil

I was truly saddened, eight years ago, when Canada Post closed the post office that was a short walk from my house. It was only a converted shop in an ugly strip of dollar stores and billiard halls, but it did somehow have a place in the community. It was the one spot where I was more than likely to bump into someone I knew. Failing that, seeing as there was almost always a line-up, it was a good chance to get to know whomever I saw. When people have time on their hands, and they are holding large parcels addressed to Ecuador or Ecum Secum, conversation is easy.

All of that stopped when they closed the post office. Friendly people were forced to look for conversation in the billiard hall, where the patrons are holding not parcels but big sticks, and where a grunt passes for oratory. The nearest post office was now too far away to be a pleasant walk, and, as a result, my efforts at correspondence, never very reliable, dwindled to near-extinction.

Then I discovered e-mail. As you will have realized by now, I'm no techno-geek, but, for me, this was a huge improvement. First of all, with e-mail, whoever gets my letter has some chance of actually being able to read it. That was seldom the case in the past. Compared to me, most medical doctors qualify as calligraphers. And, more important, with e-mail there is a much greater likelihood that I will get around to writing at all. There is something about a bale-of-hay-sized pile of letters, all waiting to be answered, that, for me, just takes the fun out of writing. I pick up the pen, I scratch out a line or two, try to say something meaningful, and half an hour later I've written three unintelligible postcards of no sentimental or even informational value, and I've still got another three hundred to go.

Once we'd bought a computer, I saw no reason ever to buy a stamp again.

Until last winter, when I stumbled on the one shining advantage the postal service still has over e-mail. When an e-mail goes astray, if it is misaddressed or somehow incorrectly routed, it has no hope. Whether it is an ardent plea of love, a highly sensitive government document or a bill for oral surgery, it's either sent unceremoniously back home or left wandering in the ether. There are many services available on the Electronic Superhighway, but compassion isn't one of them.

Not so, I found out, at Canada Post. Deliveries might be slow, strikes all too frequent and the service disgruntled and awful, but, somewhere deep in the system, there is a place that cares.

One day last winter, a letter arrived at the CBC from a woman named Anne. She lived just north of Toronto. "Please send me the recipe for Seville Orange Marmalade that aired on your program on February 1, '97," her letter said, and it was signed with a thank you. This was absolutely not out of the ordinary. "Fresh Air," the show in question, has been offering all kinds of information like that through the mail for years. Now and then a listener who requested information on a book nominated for the Giller Prize has received something on the history of porridge, but that can hardly be considered the fault of the postal system.

Anne's letter was not in good shape. The paper it was written on smelled of smoke, the envelope had burn marks on it, and the whole thing was delivered to us inside a plastic bag, inside another envelope from Canada Post. There was a form letter, too. It came from the Customer Service Department. It said Anne's letter had been violated or burned by persons unknown, and there was a number to call.

I called.

I didn't learn a whole lot right away, except that the people who work for Canada Post get very nervous when you tell them you work for a radio station. They asked why I was calling and what I was going to do with the information. They put me on hold for a very long time, and then they told me to call the Media Relations Office.

I wasn't sure what they had to hide. I mean, Anne's letter *did* arrive. It wasn't even noticeably late. If she'd been reporting a spy ring, for example, or providing the missing piece in an ongoing investigation of white-collar crime . . . but a marmalade recipe? What were they so steamed up about?

Eventually some facts came to light. Chris, from the Media Relations Office at Canada Post, called me back and told me there had been a fire. Somebody had dropped something—a cigarette, perhaps—into a mailbox on a Saturday night, and Anne's letter, along with her stamped, self-addressed envelope, had ended up in the middle of a blazing inferno so hot it warped the mailbox. The fire department had to pry it open with a crowbar. It took several gallons of water to put the fire out.

Then, Chris told me, the police department took the box and all that was left of the mail, which turned out to be 250 pieces, downtown to the police station until Monday morning, when it was all sent to the UMO.

"The UMO?" I asked.

Undeliverable Mail Office.

"Oh," I said. "Where *is* the UMO?"

He wouldn't tell me. I asked him why not, and, well, he wouldn't really tell me that, either. But he gave me Denise's number. She's a supervisor at the UMO. At least, that's what she said she was. I was beginning to wonder. She was not exactly what you'd call forthcoming.

The more they tried to withhold information about the UMO, the clearer my own imaginary picture of the place began to be. To my mind, it has to be a bit of a sanctuary. Letters are very personal things. The writer has to sit down and think about who he's writing to. He has to search for just the words he needs to tell that person what is on his mind, and the piece of paper he writes on and sends is the sole vehicle for all of that effort and expression. A lost letter, then, is like a lost soul. It doesn't know where it came from. It has a vague notion of where it is going, but nothing is very clear, and unless it gets there, those precious thoughts never leave the page.

I pictured the careful Canada Post employees that were lucky enough to be chosen to work at the UMO. There are thirty-six of them, I found out. They're the only people in Canada who can legally open mail that isn't addressed to them.

I imagine, for instance, the letter that might come from the widower who has decided, after ten years of living alone, that maybe it's time he found out what happened to that woman he met on the train before he was married. But the address is old, she hasn't lived there for years, and the building's been torn down. And because he's nervous about writing after, what is it, forty-three years? he forgets to put on a return address. That's okay. His letter is rescued by the UMO.

I asked Denise if that kind of thing did happen. She wouldn't confirm or deny it. But she did tell me a few things.

They get millions and millions of letters and parcels every year, and about 85 percent of them eventually find their way to where they were supposed to go. With the remaining 15 percent, two things can happen. Some of it is destroyed—guns, bullets and booze, for instance. Lots of booze, actually. You can't send alcohol by the mail in Canada. Well, you can, but if you do it goes to the UMO, and they pour it down the drain. The rest of that 15 percent gets sent to Crown Assets and put up for auction.

I asked Denise what they'd sent off to auction recently.

"Dolls," she said. "Pictures, a lobster cage and a tire."

"What kind of tire?" I asked.

A truck tire, as it happens. The big kind they use on large construction vehicles, and on those off-road monster trucks built to get through anything. It went into the ditch at Canada Post, and not even the UMO could get it back on the road.

It occurred to me that there probably weren't *that* many people in Canada sending giant truck tires through the mail, and that if the people at the UMO weren't quite so secretive about themselves, and where they work, they could make their jobs a little easier.

"We're not secretive," Denise said. Then she put me on hold again.

But I guess I could see their point of view, too. Truck tires are one thing, but if Canada Post put up a notice asking whoever it was that sent the $20,000 in numbered bills through the mail last week to come to such and such address and retrieve it, things might get complicated.

And besides, most of the time, the UMO gets its job done just fine. When it came to Anne's letter asking for our marmalade recipe, they were right on. It was dry, legible, as clean as could be reasonably expected and only a few days late. There were even a few Seville oranges still around in the markets, so Anne still had a chance to make her marmalade when she received the recipe she asked for. I never heard back from her, so I assume she got my letter. After all, I sent it in the mail.

Garbage and Ageage

I've already admitted to a latent nostalgia for old gear, but I wouldn't want that to be confused with any sentimentality for garbage. Where I come from, garbage is garbage. It belongs on the curb, and in my house, I'm the one who puts it there. It's a guy thing, I know. As a nod to my forefathers-in-trash, I take it seriously. And it *is* serious. These days, like manliness itself, garbage is complicated.

When I take out the trash I have to separate the paper for recycling, the cans and bottles, too, and lately, the plastic containers. (In Toronto, where I live, the system can handle the plastic with a number one or two in the little logo on the bottom, but not the threes, fours or fives.) There is also compost to deal with, and garden waste to be set out on the appropriate day (every second Monday in the spring and fall). There are even two or three days in early January set aside for retired Christmas trees.

I'm not complaining about this. Today's garbage is obviously demanding that its handlers become more environmentally responsible, and the task, for the most part, is still well within my inherited trash-slinging skills. The trouble is, lately, it seems that sometimes garbage *isn't* garbage. In fact, it's getting harder to figure out exactly what belongs on the curb.

For my dad, everything under the lid was garbage. Once we'd stuffed it in, no matter what it was, it was gone, and nobody wanted to see it again. Not surprisingly, after a few decades of that kind of thinking, cities started running out of room at the dump. So, they asked people to cut down a little bit, to take off the lid and see what they could find.

What they found—at least, a few of the smart ones—was money.

When the City of Toronto began its paper recycling program (every second Tuesday on my street), it wasn't just helping me keep the house neat. Recycled paper stock made money for them. Lots of money.

Don't get me wrong, I don't want it back—especially not the Sears flyers with the pictures of Gordie Howe in them. But the point is, had I wanted some of that paper back (a Victoria's Secret catalogue, perhaps) I would probably have had to pay for it, and that, to me, means it wasn't garbage any more.

I've struggled for a word that describes what it became. Paraphernalia is too fanciful. Matter is too scientific, and it brings up anti-matter, which, in this equation, would be the garbage, thus making my weekly trash assignment not only thought-provoking but life-threatening. Manliness has its limits. So, after some deliberation, and with both apologies and credit to George Carlin, I'm calling it *stuff*. And the difference, in my little thesis, between stuff and garbage has to do with age and money.

I once met an archaeologist named Ed Keall, who

worked with the Royal Ontario Museum. Ed was involved in a dig in Zabid, Yemen. There is a citadel there that flourished under the Ottoman Empire in the fourteenth and fifteenth centuries. The history of the city itself goes back much further than that. Ed has found a number of artifacts from the twelfth century, and even some from the ninth. Some of those came from the kitchens they'd unearthed, and other public areas in the city, but the best source of accurate historical information, Ed told me, was the latrine.

And that was mostly, if you'll excuse me, because of the chunks. The pieces of glass and pottery they found in the latrines were just plain bigger than the stuff they found anywhere else.

Ed Keall's explanation was partly that, in some cases, the latrine might have been used as a general purpose garbage can. But, more likely, if something was in the outhouse, it was because somebody wanted it to stay there. When the mixing bowl that was a wedding present from Uncle Ahmed finally gave up the ghost after years of noble service, it wasn't surreptitiously chucked. It was given a proud parade at the top of the barrow all the way to the dump. But when the brand new gravy boat Mom ordered from the catalogue store in Constantinople took a ding in the spout from nine-year-old Nuri, who was using it as a battleship playing Turks and Greeks out in the breezeway, that gravy boat went to the bottom of the blackest of Black Seas, where no one would ever find it, or even think of looking, especially Mom.

Then, when an archaeologist finds that gravy boat and gets very excited, that gravy boat is no longer garbage. It is something a museum wants and will pay great piles of money to have. It is now stuff. Very good stuff, in fact. It is encased in glass, expertly lit and tended to with great care by archaeological experts of every stripe, and millions of paying museum patrons line up to see it every year.

Age and money.

The gravy boat story is a good one for my purposes, and not only because it covers great stretches of time and ends with great piles of money. In the case of the gravy boat there is never any question about whose it was. Little Nuri didn't want it back, and even if his mother did, she wouldn't have been willing to do anything about it. For stuff belonging to humans, generally speaking, the trip to the outhouse is final. People do not think "What the heck?" and leap into the cesspool on the off chance that they might find the missing gravy boat, or their watch, or even their wedding rings. Ed Keall told me they find astounding amounts of obviously very precious jewellery in latrine sites, but very little in the way of human remains, and certainly none wearing bathing trunks or snorkels. People just aren't willing to go in there, for anything. Which means whatever fell in isn't theirs any more.

We've evolved a legal system of patent and trademark registration, pre-nuptial agreements and litigious actions of every description, but the true and final measure of who gets to keep what is still the schoolyard bully's tried and true question. "Hey!" you yell at the privy. "That's my wedding ring!" "Yeah?" gurgles back an ominous voice. "What are you going to do about it?"

End of story.

So, when trying to determine whether a given object is stuff or garbage, where it lies is at least as important as what it is. A cherished gravy boat in a latrine is garbage, at least for the first nine hundred years. A cherished item—let's say a book, left at a friend's place—even though it is no longer in the possession of the original owner, is still very much stuff, perhaps even, one could argue, still the original owner's stuff, even if the friend throws it out.

If the book in question is this one, I'll vouch for you, if you still want it back. Failing that, ask your friend to leave it in an outhouse. If nobody reads it, or, more likely, when the next person to read it gets to this point (or before) nine hundred years from now, you will have done my descendants a favour.

Or not.

Anyway, those are the two extremes, as I see them: the outhouse bully at one end, and your copy of *King Lear* (it's just clearer this way) left at a friend's at the other. And if I could be permitted a small review of the equation (as much for my elucidation as for yours), so far, it goes like this:

There's garbage and there's stuff. All garbage starts out as stuff (the gravy boat before the accident), until, eventually, it becomes garbage (if Nuri hadn't busted it something else would have).

Therefore: Stuff + Age = Garbage

But if it stays garbage long enough (e.g., nine hundred years), it becomes stuff again.

So: Garbage + Age = Stuff

Are you still with me? If not, and you're thinking you'll throw this down the outhouse to see if it looks any better in nine hundred years, don't do it yet. There's another factor in all of this. It has to do with what happened when recycled paper pulled that neat little trick of turning from garbage into stuff when money came along.[1] There are other ways that garbage can turn into stuff, but I'll warn you now, they are considerably less pretty than a pile of old lingerie catalogues.

Fair Toronto, on whose curbs I have been leaving my former stuff for the past ten years, has already stuffed one landfill site to bulging. The Brock West landfill site closed in late October 1996 after taking in a whopping 282,587 tonnes of trash. The other site the city operates, Keele Valley, opened in 1983, and was, until recently, to close in 2002, with a projected total of 1,515,158 tonnes. They are now thinking they'll let that pile get even heavier.

But the reason it's closing isn't the weight of the trash, it's the size. The Keele Valley site is a former gravel pit. It's about one kilometre wide and thirty metres deep, but they're going to pile the trash up another twenty metres or so before they close it.

Think of the highest diving board used in Olympic competition. The ten-metre board is so high you can think of several very long biblical verses before you hit the water and recite them all. Well, if you were diving from the top of the almost-mile-wide pile of garbage at Keele Valley, you'd be five times that high, about as tall as a seventeen-storey building.

---

[1] I feel obliged to tell you, at this point, that here in Toronto, the selling of recycled paper has now turned out to be, I'm sorry to say, not quite as lucrative as it once was. Although the city is still collecting my paper for recycling, they're not getting as much money for it as they once were. Some reports say they're not getting any money at all. Apparently, once it became clear that old paper was worth something, the supply quickly outweighed the demand, resulting in far more newsprint than was fit to recycle. But, as you'll see, that doesn't mean it went back to being garbage.

And speaking of high, don't forget your nose-plugs. A by-product of the Keele Valley landfill site, aside from close to one hundred full-time jobs, is ten million cubic feet of methane every day.

But it is precisely those charming features that, for at least one enterprising outfit, have turned Toronto's garbage into stuff. You see, that great square pile of trash is so huge and so foul that we have to pay someone else to deal with it. As of January 1998, Browning-Ferris Industries (BFI) has a three-year contract to remove about 20 percent of our solid waste (we're keeping the methane for ourselves) to its corporate home in Auburn Hills, Michigan. That's forty tractor-trailer loads of Toronto's Finest every day, lumbering down Highway 401 and across the border into the amber waves of grain.

And those American trade negotiators accuse us of dumping! There probably *will* be a few pounds of Pacific salmon or softwood lumber in there. But the Americans don't have anything to complain about here. BFI is getting fifty-three dollars per tonne out of the deal, for a minimum of 250,000 tonnes. You can do the math yourself. It's more than enough to buy a new gravy boat.

To Browning-Ferris Industries, those forty tractor-trailer loads are not garbage. They are BFI's reason for being. Okay, once it gets to Auburn Hills, Michigan, BFI is going to burn it or bury it or build a subdivision over it or something equally dismissive, but still, they are driving four hours each way to get that trash. They want it. To them, because of the money involved, it's not garbage, it's stuff.

So: Garbage (no matter how foul or how much) + Money = Stuff

This is where my father-in-law comes in.

Eric, my father-in-law, has no trouble seeing stuff in his garbage. For Eric, a successful trip to the dump isn't measured by what you leave behind but by what you bring back. Eric lives in Toronto, but his favourite dump is the one closest to the family cottage, about three hours north. At one point, he was going so often we started calling it "the Mall."

At first I thought of Eric as somewhat of an oddity. Well, let's be honest: I couldn't believe that somehow, just because I was inexorably drawn to his daughter, I suddenly had to count him as family. For me, raised as a keep-the-lid-on-the-can, manly garbage-handler, who wouldn't think of going to the dump except perhaps to give them tips on how they could heave more of it down that hole, and faster, Eric wasn't just an oddity, he was a freak.

After asking around a bit, though, I found he wasn't the only one to use the dump as more of a lending library than a permanent repository. When I was speaking to a group of Lutherans in Don Mills on this topic (it's true), I met a couple who used the word "dump" as a verb, as in "We're going dumping this weekend," which, of course, meant precisely the opposite.

Another person I found, shopping in a town not far from one of the Lutherans' favourite spots, was referred to the dump by a local retailer. She needed a stove rack, and she'd looked in every store in town to absolutely no avail. Finally, in Stedman's, while the manager was rooting around the supply room, one of the cashiers pulled her aside and whispered, "Why don't you just go to the dump? There are five or six of them there, behind the dumpster. No one's going to know."

She did go, and she found one right away. More important, she stayed for half an hour and has since gone back several times, sometimes just to watch the bears.

But perhaps it is unfair to introduce Eric along with this crowd. Perhaps, without greater establishment of my father-in-law's character in this story, I will find myself without a seat, let alone my usual serving of pumpkin pie, at Thanksgiving dinner this year.

First of all, Eric grew up in Newfoundland in the leanest time this century has known. Things were not thrown out in Newfoundland in the 1930s and '40s—not food, not clothing, not even ideas of debatable value, such as union with Canada. I grew up in Canada's then most powerful economic centre (Montreal) in an era of prosperity (the 1960s and '70s) in which everything—food, clothing, brassieres, big bands, the English language, the supremacy of the Catholic Church, vast numbers of ideas (almost including union with Canada) and, ultimately, even the state of being the economic centre of power—was thrown out, mostly to a landfill site called Toronto, about five hours to the west along Highway 401. It is possible Eric considered picking those things up, and, if he couldn't use them, selling them in a garage sale.

Around here, you don't have to be a Michigan-based waste dealer earning $13,250,000 (I knew you wouldn't do the math) to be in on the business of turning garbage into stuff. There is a network of garbage retrieval, sale and resale in this city—a Brown Market, if you will—that, to me, anyway, defies belief.

One man up the street from us specializes in the salvage resale of zippers. Not clothing, just zippers. His property is festooned with them, drooping and grotesque, like an explosion of garment entrails, every Saturday morning. Another fellow in the neighbourhood deals solely in kites, many of them still soiled from their brush with the dump (something that could be, I suppose, referred to as a "malling"). There is the corrugated-fibre-glass-bits man, the toilet-seat man, several dozen hubcap men, the lawnmower man . . . Each Saturday they cover their lawns with what a lot of the rest of us, but obviously not all of us, would consider garbage, and they wait for like-minded souls to duke it out for the spot at the top of the haggling heap, reserved for the one who will least budge from what is arbitrarily deemed a fair price.

And these guys are tough. It's easier arguing with a bank teller over service charges. I once tangled with the lawnmower man over an electric, twin-blade, fully functional model I had lying around the garage. Okay, yes, I had more than one. All right, I had three, and I go to the Mall a lot now, too. The best time is sundown. It's nice.

Anyway, I wanted five bucks for the lawnmower. Five bucks! It worked perfectly well. I'd already brought it to him. I wheeled it forward, running the gauntlet of his overpriced mowers all the way up the front walk, and he, the lawnmower man, without looking, said, "Dollar-fifty."

I displayed its features, which, granted, didn't take long, but I thought I did a good job. I plugged it in. *I mowed his lawn*. He didn't blink. I fumed, I ranted. Nothing. I stalked back down the front walk, disgraced because I still had the damn lawnmower that I didn't want, and no five bucks, or even dollar-fifty, which, truth be told, by that point I would have liked, because it was hot, and the corner store was right there, full of Popsicles. The lawnmower man, however, continued to ignore me and even went back to reading his book (which, for all I know, was my copy of *King Lear*).

In short, I lost. I failed to turn my lawnmower from garbage into stuff. In fact, in order to finally get rid of it, I gave it away. My dad has it now. He likes it fine. I've even considered inviting him to the Mall.

Anyway, the way I look at it is this: everything is garbage until somebody wants it, and then it becomes stuff, which they will eventually want to throw out, at which point it will be garbage again, until someone else wants it, and it once again becomes stuff, unless there is money involved, in which case, if a person has to pay to be rid of their stuff, it becomes garbage to the ridder and stuff to the riddee, unless it is thrown in an outhouse, which will render it garbage, regardless of intrinsic value, for a very long time, until somebody working for a museum finds it, at which point it will be stuff once again and worth far more money than it ever was before.

Or: Stuff + Age = Garbage
Garbage + Age = Stuff
Garbage + Money = Stuff

And, then, logically:
Stuff + Money = Garbage

Therefore:
Age = Money

So, if you are looking at a pile of stuff somewhere in your place and wondering what to pitch and what to keep, go get yourself a beer and see what's on the Garbage

Channel (last I checked there were several of them), because the only way to sort it out is to wait a good, long time.

And, if it is now the year 2897, and you are an archaeologist at a latrine site, hoping for the big discovery that's going to net you piles of cash and fame and academic credibility and give you a glittering artifact that the museum back home will gladly display with great prominence for all of its millions of visitors to enjoy for centuries to come, and instead you've found this book, I'm sorry.

But if you keep digging, past the lawnmower, and the other lawnmower, and the 1,515,158 tonnes of late-twentieth-century Canadian urban trash, and the English language, and the supremacy of the Catholic Church in Quebec, and the twelfth-century gravy boat, you might find something really valuable. I just know it's there. I had it in my hand only minutes ago. It's my copy of *King Lear*.

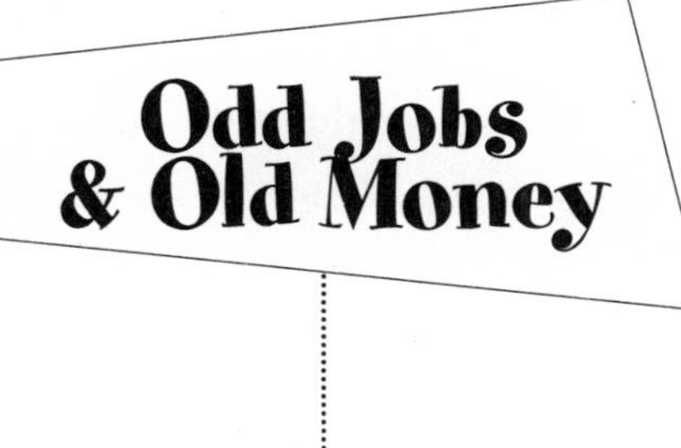

I hardly look at my paycheque any more. Every two weeks it gets blipped into my account by invisible electronic gremlins and, within the next two weeks, it is blipped back out by equally mysterious forces. Theoretically I know that money is what provides me and my family with a roof, a car, food and clothes. When I look at the numbers on that stub of paper that I bring home from work I know that, by any rational standard, I am truly a wealthy man. But in the steps of my daily life, it seems to me that the more I make, the less I have.

That's why, lately, I've been thinking fondly of the luxurious days before I had any money.

For six years after I graduated from university, if anyone asked, I said I was a musician. It was true. I even played, truth be told, a couple of gigs that were legitimately impressive. But if I were to add up all of my gigs in those six years, including the ones I told no one about then and certainly won't admit to here, it would probably amount to only about eighteen months' worth of work.

The rest of the time I was a secretary. I worked as a temp. Bear in mind that this was in New York during the boom years of the late 1980s, when a person could get full-time work as a pollster by claiming to have watched "Family Feud." My qualifications for the title of "secretary"—let alone "legal secretary"—were shaky at best. I started as a receptionist at the legal firm of Obermeyer, Morvillo & Abramowitz. My job was to answer the phone, which, considering that I had to say "Obermeyer, Morvillo & Abramowitz," with a smile, about five hundred times every day, was no picnic. But it left plenty of time between calls to teach myself to type.

Once I could bang out a memo in less time than it took for the lawyers to start yelling, I got hired as a word-processor with the HongKong Bank, and I knew I'd hit the jackpot. The work was easy, they paid me more than twice what I'd earned as a receptionist, and, when the phone rang, I only had to say three syllables instead of twelve. When I moved to Toronto I found almost limitless demand for my secretarial services with the big Bay Street law firms, and, to my astonishment, they were also willing to pay what seemed to me to be vast amounts of money.

Of course, it wasn't. At the time I was sharing a house with an engineer who'd been gainfully employed for about ten years. One spring, while I was doing my tax return, curiosity got the better of him and he asked what I made. He had to ask me a second time. Then he bought me dinner.

But in the luxury department, I was loaded.

There was a cheese shop down the street, right next to a bakery. The law firm was so frantic with work that if I called to say I'd be late no one wasted any time asking why. So, on sunny mornings in May and June, and there were plenty, I would assemble my vast sums of spare cash and buy a pound of ridiculously expensive coffee, a bag of fresh crusty rolls and, from the cheese shop, a wedge of what I now realize, for me, will be the substance of the very steps to Heaven: fresh, fragrant, flaky Asiago cheese.

Back home on the porch, with the city abuzz around me, I felt every bit the wealthy sophisticate who could ask nothing more of life than that it stay the way it was for just a little longer.

It didn't. Within a year I was engaged to be married and began having conversations with real estate agents. Within five years I was a husband, father and homeowner, living at the opposite end of town from the cheese shop, which had gone out of business. And now, ten years later, when I wade through the nightmare that my tax return has become, I have to fight to think of those mornings simply as they were, instead of calculating how much more spare change I would now have if I had worked through those mornings, foregone the cheese and coffee and invested the proceeds in an RRSP.

My only hope is that for the next ten or twenty years

this pattern will continue. If so, my insurance costs will become staggering, my children exorbitant, my retirement investments voracious, and my salary, no matter what it is, will be absolutely consumed without a trace, until I am downsized and sent home with no money at all.

With any luck, that will happen just after I've run out of things to spend it on, and I will be left looking for some small amount of work to help me get by, perhaps as a receptionist who can speak twelve syllables with a smile.

With any luck, it will be in May, or June, and my mornings will be unspoken for.

With even more luck, even if none of that comes to be, the steps to Heaven *will* be made of Asiago cheese. I just hope the coffee is strong enough, too.

Pay Now, Live Later

I was but a lad when I first apprenticed in the art of the investment. My twelve-year-old sister, Denise, was my teacher, and our boardroom was the back seat of our family's 1968 Dodge Polara. We were rattling through the secondary roads of New England on the way to Maine for a family camping trip. I was nine. I was hungry. I'd eaten both the candies Mom had given me not one minute earlier and was busy licking my palms for any remaining residue. Denise still had both of hers. She was admiring their cellophane wrappers.

"See the way the stripe goes all the way around and starts on the other side?" she said, turning each one slowly.

I began to sweat.

Two hours later, and at least five times through the local radio station's heavy rotation of "Hand Me Down World" by the Guess Who, she had almost finished her first candy, and I was bargaining for her second. I'd already offered her the grape soda I was gambling I could get at our next stop, half of all my candy from the tuck shop in the first week of our holiday and an ice cream at the Sealtest Dairy when we got back home.

She was thinking about it.

When I finally got the candy, it was the only one I was going to eat on the entire trip. And when I opened it, I found it was the kind with the green stripes, not the red. These were far inferior in my opinion, an opinion, I then gathered from the look on Denise's face, of which my sister had been ruthlessly aware all along.

But by the time we got to Maine she'd already forgotten the whole deal. After writing out the now considerable portfolio of bonbon bonds that I had agreed to provide, and reading and rereading the list for hours on a hot day, in the back seat of a late-model Dodge on secondary roads, she barfed, and cleared her memory banks, as well as her stomach, of all things edible. I went on to eat as much candy as I could have wanted that holiday, including several packages of butter toffee, which eventually made me sick, too. Our relationship has remained peaceable ever since.

There you have it: supply, demand, price gouging, the futures market, market correction due to overwhelming internal forces and, rare in an investment story, a happy ending.

And that *is* what matters most in an investment story: the ending. It is, after all, the rainy day we're all saving for, even though most investors are loath to admit it. As loath, certainly, as the people who want them to buy investments. Death is not a popular topic in the investment community. I may yet see an RRSP advertisement showing a dull, old, drooling man in a wheelchair bumping his gums about how glad he is to still have enough money for Jell-O, but I'm not going to hold my breath. Neither should he. Especially if he's going to be selling RRSPs. Any actor who is going to get a part flogging RRSPs has to be able to pull his weight in a rowing scull with a bunch of Ivy League cadets, sail a sloop around the Cape of Good Hope or at least sprint through the financial district in an Armani pinstripe suit.

I knew a couple in Montreal who got dressed up to run places. They were students, with little reason to don business attire and less reason to run. But they felt while running—a young, handsome couple, meeting life with trench coats open and hair blown back—that they looked as if they had exciting lives. In fact, their lives consisted of going to class, studying and visiting their parents. Aside from their duplicitous jogs through town, if they were dressed up, it was for a roast dinner at Mom's, and if they were running, it was to get there before the Yorkshire pudding fell.

I have since lost track of them. But I feel sure they will live for a good, long time and die fabulously wealthy. Because, at twenty-one, they were relentlessly earnest and careful to make only exactly the right choices in life—just the types to buy the idea that by putting away little bits of money early on they might end up rowing with the Ivy Leaguers and sailing sloops around the Cape of Good Hope.

That's the hard part for me. For people who are actually engaged in the business of *living*, the idea of saving for old age doesn't settle in until young age has already moved out and is running down the street in an open trench coat. And it's not coming back for dinner, either.

Perhaps you've already ascertained my own personal stake in this story. Yes, my sister taught me as much as she could about buying low, selling high and hanging on to your assets, if not your cookies, in a volatile market. But it still wasn't enough to get my face out of the candy wrapper in time to do anything about it.

The first clue I had that I had already missed the investing sloop (no matter where it was headed) was a subway ad featuring Janie and Willy. You probably saw it too. The names change every RRSP season, but the story is the same. Janie, at twenty-one, puts a small chunk into an RRSP every month for ten years, and then stops. Willy, at thirty-one, puts the same amount in every month, and does so for thirty-four years, after which time he still has less than Janie.

How does this work? It's called compound interest, and it's very easy to explain. First of all, at age twenty-one, Janie is as dull as hardwood floors in a salt factory. She has no interest at all in her life, except for the kind that comes from a bank, which she reinvests until she's sixty-five, when she cashes it all in for one big spree. Willy, on the other hand, has a youth that is so interesting he has to be put *in* a compound, until he turns sixty-five and is released with no money. But since he has to find work, he gets a job piloting a sloop around the Cape of Good Hope, which is, coincidentally, the same one Janie has hired for her big spree. Then they are struck by a rowing scull full of investment bankers and everybody dies.

I told you happy endings were rare. Especially with an ad campaign aimed at twenty-one-year-olds that is read only by thirty-one-year-olds. What twenty-one-year-old thinks about retiring? These days most of them are still thinking about finding work.

Now, if Kurt Winter had made an ad for RRSPs, I'd be rich today.

Kurt Winter was a big, hairy rock 'n' roll guitarist from

Winnipeg who could write, sing and burn out searing solos that would take the barnacles right off your sloop. In 1970 he was driving a car that had "a milk carton for a carburetor" and playing with a trio called Brother, with drummer Vance Masters and bassist Bill Wallace. Brother is still legendary in local music circles, but they were by no means a safe investment. They doggedly played original music in a market that would pay only for pop covers, and they generally thumbed their noses at the entire music establishment.

Then, on a May weekend in 1970, with one phone call, Kurt Winter *became* the music establishment. That weekend another Winnipeg-based band found itself without a guitarist and asked Kurt to join, along with fellow Winnipegger Greg Liskew. The Guess Who had a huge hit single on the charts, their fifth gold record in two years, a number-one album and another recording date already booked. Mere weeks after Kurt joined, the band opened a concert for forty thousand people in Montreal with his song "Hand Me Down World," soon to be enjoyed on back roads all over North America. A few days after the concert in Montreal, as a member of the Guess Who, Kurt Winter was performing at the White House for President Richard Nixon, his daughter Tricia and Prince Charles and Princess Anne. The group outsold all other music groups in singles sales in 1970, including the Beatles, and made more than $2 million, with earnings on outstanding royalties projected at $5 million for 1971.

None of that seemed to change Kurt's lifestyle much. His wardrobe, for example, stayed exactly the same from the time he stuffed it into a paper bag on his way out of Winnipeg to join the band. It consisted of one pair of green-and-white striped pants and (possibly) two "Sound by Garnet" sweatshirts, with sleeves cut off at the shoulder. You can see Kurt's wardrobe on the cover of the band's 1970 *Share the Land* album. You can also see it on the cover of *The Best of the Guess Who* (1971) and *So Long Bannatyne* (1971), *Rockin'* (1972), *Live at the Paramount* (1972) and *Artificial Paradise* (1973), by which time he'd changed the pants.

Given that he didn't spend much on clothes, you might well wonder what he did with all the money. A certain amount was, to be sure, spent on what might be politely deemed "hedonistic recreation." But still, how much money can you spend on pizza and drugs in a matter of months? "Hand Me Down World," credited solely to Kurt as composer, reached number 17 on the U.S. charts, number 10 in Canada, and sold over 900,000 copies. Exact figures are hard to come by, but he was doing all right.

He did buy a white Cadillac, and a house on working-class Chevrier Boulevard in Winnipeg. In John Einarson's 1995 book *American Woman*, Kurt said: "I didn't change anything else. I ate better food, but I didn't go extravagant. I was always used to living in some dungeon and now I finally had a back yard I could go out and piss in."

If the Guess Who didn't wear suits, they weren't against hiring them. At some point in their flurry of fortune they took on a Winnipeg financial adviser, who paid them each a limited salary (protection from the tax man) and funnelled the rest into part ownership of a shopping mall in Red Deer, Alberta, a hotel in Jamaica, some prime Winnipeg real estate and a series of Kentucky Fried Chicken outlets in the United States.

Kurt stayed with the band for four years. Then, after

endless touring, drinking, smoking, eating, a certain amount of groupie indulgence, eight albums and dozens of songs, the others asked him to leave because he was too plowed to bother showing up at the recording sessions any more.

Still, in those four years, he'd generated a fantastic amount of revenue. Exactly how much will likely remain a mystery. By the time the band finally folded, a year or so after Kurt left, the books were a complete mess and Revenue Canada was all over them like a dirty "Sound by Garnet" sweatshirt.

The trusted financial advisers, it turned out, shouldn't have been. The shopping mall had gone into receivership. The Winnipeg real estate lost value. The fast-food outlets were poorly managed. There were all kinds of questionable entries on the ledger, including the expenses of a failed travel agency for the band's record label, management's bad debts covered by the band's personal accounts and, inexplicably, the purchase of some canoes for a summer camp.

One former band member who had been with the group since the very beginning had to sell his house, his art collection and his Mercedes-Benz just to pay the back taxes. After that he took a job as a hotel clerk to make ends meet.

Kurt hung on to his back yard to piss in, but not much else. "After all the money we'd made and all the crap I went through," he said in Einarson's book, "I got $25,000; $10,000 went to my accountant and $15,000 went to my lawyer, and I got zip."

Not exactly a happy ending, either, I know. But, in a sense, Kurt backed the right horse. It's difficult to imagine him doing anything but what he did during his youth. Even our Janie might have given up on her monthly instalments to fly around the world playing to millions of fans and living like rock 'n' roll royalty. For Kurt, there surely must have been few regrets. He died in December 1997, at age fifty-three, from a stomach condition. He never needed all those investments, anyway. He had his house, his dirty sweatshirts, and he never ran out of beer. All told, he spent twenty-six years dreaming up his ideal life, four years living it, and the rest cruising to the finish line.

I bought my first Guess Who record when I was ten. Of course, Kurt wasn't shilling RRSPS on the inner sleeve. Those pants just wouldn't *do* on a sloop, and no rowing team at all concerned with staying afloat would have let him anywhere near the boathouse, let alone in the scull. But that's the point. I didn't care about that. I just wanted to be like Kurt, regardless of what he was wearing. If Kurt *had* said investing was cool, you couldn't have kept me from the bank. By the time I'd realized he was lying, he would have been dead, anyway.

And, as for me . . . Well, let's see. *The Best of the Guess Who* cost me five bucks at Steve's Record Store at the Côte-St-Luc Shopping Centre in March 1971, and *Share the Land* cost me another five the week after that. So, if I had taken ten dollars every month, invested it at an average interest rate of 10 percent until March 1977,[1] I would

---

[1] That's a year and a half after the Guess Who played their final gig at the Montreal Forum. I figure that's enough time for the fund to have turned to Disco Debt Bonds and Saturday Night Futures. By then, of course, Kurt was long gone back to Winnipeg, happily drinking beer and enjoying his yard.

have come out with an investment principal of $926, perpetually Rock 'n' Rolling over in the Fun, Fun, Fund ('Til Her Daddy Takes the T-Bills Away). The marketing possibilities are staggering. So, when I'm twenty-one, and thinking seriously about nothing for at least ten years, I've got $1,491 in the bank. At thirty-one, it's $3,868. Today, at thirty-seven, it would be $6,852. At fifty-three, the age Kurt left the life stage for good, I'll have $31,485, and, when I die at...

Well, that's the question, isn't it? I mean, if you're saving for a rainy day, it might be nice to know if there's even a low pressure zone on the way.

I've done the average numbers. They aren't indexed for lifestyle, but they still pack a punch.

As of 1994, the average life expectancy in Canada was eighty-one for women, seventy-five for men, and it's going up all the time. If the current rate of change remains constant, by the time I get to seventy-five, the average Canadian man will be living to eighty-six. That doesn't sound too bad to me. I had about twenty years of freedom at the beginning. It'll make a nice frame.

But, given the same rate of change, by the time my son retires, the average life expectancy of a Canadian man will be ninety-five. If I'm lucky enough to have a grandson to sit on my knee, when that little gaffer is ready to retire, men will be living to a hundred and three. And that won't be old, it will be the average. The old ones will be living to a hundred and forty! What are people going to do? The Kurt Winters of the future will have to stay on the road for fifty years just to afford the privilege of dying young.

As to when the buying of RRSPS will have to start, rock

stars shilling to nine-year-olds will have long missed the boat. Forget about a carefree childhood. Baby shower gifts will have to come in boxes marked Fisher Price Waterhouse. And, with kids leaving home later all the time and staying longer in school, that poor grandson of mine will graduate middle-aged, work for a few months and save like a demon so he can play shuffleboard for eighty-five years on the family team with his great-great-grandson, who will be just about ready to retire.

Forget "life management skills." "Post-career planning" will be what gets a person through.

I have an idea about this. Remember the James Cameron movie *Terminator*? Arnold Schwarzenegger (rumoured to be Hollywood's wealthiest star, and a crashing bore in his twenties, but don't tell him I said so) plays one very bad next-century robot who comes back (and back) through time to settle a very old debt. It's a great movie—terrifying and relentless. But what interests me is how it showed the world through Arnie's eyes: anytime he looked at anything he received a little readout from his internal computer, like a menu bar on the inside of his sunglasses. If he looked at a fellow outside a biker joint, for example, it told him how much the biker weighed, how powerful his bike was, how long it would take Arnie to clobber him and steal his clothes . . . that kind of stuff.

Well, in my lifetime (as yet statistically average) I have seen computers go from awkward, card-swallowing dinosaurs to wondrous machines capable of new technological feats every few weeks. How far off can Arnie's readout be? It could sample our vital signs on an ongoing basis, calculate our chances for success at a given challenge (sailing, rowing . . . you know) and access our central

DNA coding to tell us approximately how much longer we might expect to live.

So, I might look at a mille-feuille in the bakery and want to eat it right away, but, just so I know where I stand, my lifetime readout will tell me how many extra pounds I'll gain by eating it, what that will do to my cholesterol levels and overall cardiac health, and show me, with each bite, how much time off the end of my stay on earth I have just cost myself.

This personal readout might also keep track of investments, so that as the number in the upper right, representing compound interest and net worth, goes up, the number in the lower left, representing overall health and remaining lifespan, goes down.

Of course, for Arnie the cyborg—and possibly for boring Janie, too—that would all be useful information to be plugged into a predictable life course. No risks, and fewer surprises. What could be better?

But for Kurt Winter—well, who's to say? I suppose if he had known he would be leaving the stage so soon Kurt might have taken things a little easier. But, then again, maybe he *did* know. Maybe that's how he could ignore the huge profits those record company execs were throwing away on rancid chicken and just be content with a back yard to piss in.

In my mind, I picture Kurt, the defender of carefree youth, doing battle with Arnie, the relentless robot of investment responsibility. We know Arnie is indestructible, but Kurt refuses to give in. He stays at him, wailing out riffs on his beat-up Stratocaster, his forehead beading with sweat and his "Sound by Garnet" shirt damp with the toil of a lifetime on the road. And when chorus after chorus of searing blues can't blow the cyborg away, Kurt looks old age square in the face and burns out of this life in a blaze of glorious feedback.

Or maybe not. Maybe years go by, until Arnie's digital readout informs him that, at the age of 141, he's just reached the 99.9th percentile in the longevity category, and he celebrates with a trip to Maine for a summer holiday. It's a little bumpy in the back seat of his Polara, and a little warm, too. More than once, as he quietly rereads his quarterly reports, the little green light in his systems monitor indicates a potential problem in the digestive area. The action centre suggests sucking on a hard candy, but, seeing as it is 2089, and he has already outlived all reasonable expectations, his candy supply, due to sub-par performance of a poorly managed bonbon bond, has long run out.

The dividing glass between the front and back seats purrs down, and the chauffeur, a ghostly presence, leans back. "Trouble, boss?" he asks.

"I'm out of candies!" Arnie roars over the noise from the radio. *Awfully loud up there*, he thinks. *Smoky, too*.

"Gee," the chauffeur says, and he digs into a special pocket sown onto the inside of his sleeveless, dirty, 1970 sweatshirt. "I just happen to have one left," he says, as he turns the heat up slightly in the back seat and accelerates into another dip.

"What'll you give me for it?"

The Work Will Wait

I've noticed something about my motivation to work these days. I seem to be learning, finally, to coast. It could be that it is blessed summer at this point, and I'm mere days from a family holiday, but I don't think that's the entire story. Like an older house that still might be worth putting a little work into, I seem to have had my electrical systems upgraded. Time was that I would slave, like a fuse, until, in a crackling flash, I burned out and had to be removed from the job and replaced. Now, closer to forty than thirty-five, I'm feeling more like a circuit breaker. Sure, I'll pop out after a hard day, but it's no big deal. Something or someone will push me back in eventually.

It makes me think about Bob MacDonald.

Bob was my first boss. He was also, I'm guessing now in retrospect, something like Property Committee Manager at our church. He was definitely important in that community, but he didn't quite fit the mould of the Presbyterian elder. The rest of them had supple hands and banker's suits. Bob was a contractor with cracked hands as square as cinder blocks and shoulders as wide as a countertop. Every couple of years he bought an old house for his family of six to live in, fixed it up, sold it and then moved them all again. By the time I met him he'd worked more hours than I had lived.

When I was fifteen, he hired me to paint the casements of the church's stained-glass windows. This meant painting hundreds of wooden strips about half an inch wide, the slats between the panes. Bob said it might be a picky job and would probably take longer than it looked.

I didn't worry too much about that. I'd painted before. When Bob said he'd come out on the first morning to show me the ropes, I indulged him.

His hands made the brush look like a Q-tip. He did the first window for me, a neat line of bright yellow all around the stained glass. He was right-handed, but if things got awkward he simply switched to his left. He made no mistakes, and the whole window took him thirty-five minutes. Then he handed me the brush, pointed me toward the next window and said goodbye.

I was still there at quitting time, eight hours later. I'd spent more time wiping glass than I had painting wood. I'd had to lean way back for so long to get at the underside of one bit that when I finally had it done I couldn't stand up. My hair had dried into the paint behind me. The church was across the street from our house. I had to yell for my mom.

But I got the hang of it over the next few weeks. By then I needed only two or three hours for each of those windows. I even started to enjoy it. I liked the feeling of purpose as I set out each morning, and, at the end of the day, there was shiny new yellow trim where peeling grey had been the day before. It was satisfying.

"There's a name for what you're feeling," my dad told

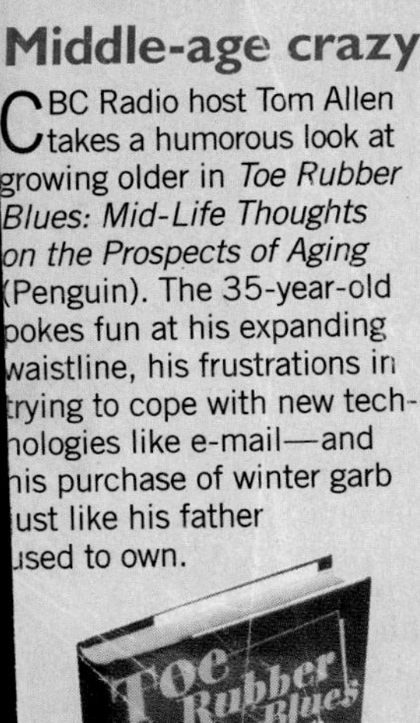
Middle-age crazy

CBC Radio host Tom Allen takes a humorous look at growing older in *Toe Rubber Blues: Mid-Life Thoughts on the Prospects of Aging* (Penguin). The 35-year-old pokes fun at his expanding waistline, his frustrations in trying to cope with new technologies like e-mail—and his purchase of winter garb just like his father used to own.

me. "It's the Protestant Work Ethic." I wondered if it was happening because I was working on a church.

As it turns out, though, the work ethic is a religion in itself, and the Protestants have long lost control of its boundaries. It is now an ecumenical sect with well-maintained missions in every branch of western life. It has multiple levels of orthodoxy, fundamentalist extremists, evangelists and even heretics that have been banished for life. And, like any system of faith, it has a few problems. It doesn't allow much room in the liturgy for family communication, for one thing, and there are a whole bunch of wonderful things that it just won't give the time of day to, like playing catch, or dancing. Daydreaming is well beyond the pale.

That was a problem for me. I could work like a demon once I'd decided a job was worth my time, but in between feverish bouts, I'd always been a daydreamer. In fact, as a painter, I had deliberately taken jobs where I knew I could zone out without getting thrown out.

It started with the job at the Scurfields'. I was fourteen. I had to strip the old paint off the ceiling of the front porch and repaint everything. It meant hours on a step ladder, back bent and arms aching, painstakingly heating the old paint with a blowtorch until it could be scraped away like pizza topping to drop in searing clumps on my face and arms. Mr. Scurfield paid me two dollars per hour for that. On my first morning of searing pizza I began to wonder if I'd been had. Until lunch time.

I'm not sure if Mr. Scurfield felt guilty about the job, or the wage, or both, but as he left for work that first day, he decided to include lunch. He showed me where the fridge was, set up a TV tray in the solarium in front of the

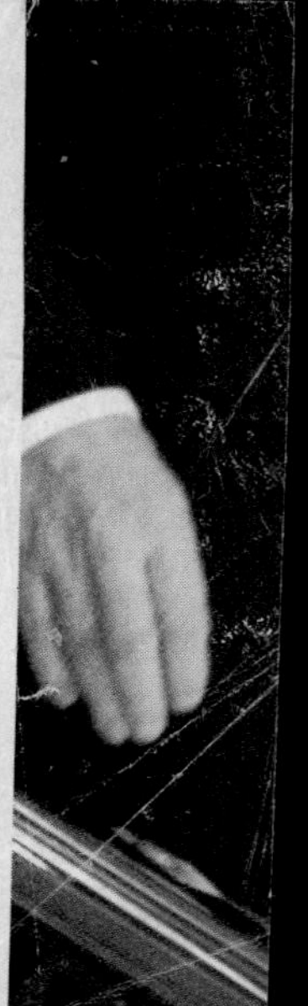

n good," his
your alarm
on the way.
xes, so take
on more to

can take to
the rhetoric
ent's critics.
rnment had
w tax cuts,
e right; not
e NDP from
high-income
x break, and
ggest the ex-
health care
lays of fiscal
out his cred-
as Canadian
ncy Hughes

ne numbers.
ed Ottawa's

La-Z-Boy and said I could help myself. I was a fourteen-year-old boy! I'd have paid *him* two dollars an hour to eat his food. And TV, too? It was too much. "The Gong Show" was on at noon. By the end of the job, the porch was pure, gleaming white, so was the inside of the fridge, and I could sing "It's Been So Lonesome In The Saddle Since My Horse Died" by heart. If this was work, and I was being ethically responsible by doing it, I knew I had found my calling.

When Bob MacDonald hired me to paint the church, I knew my days of daydreaming destiny had finally come.

I had my own key to the place. If I had done my work quickly enough to be ahead of schedule, or if it was raining, I honestly had nothing else to do but go inside.

There were all kinds of odd little corners and hidden staircases in that church. I can still smell the wood in the study, and in the choir room there was an old electric organ. No one was ever around in that church in the summertime. I could go in there and play the organ anytime I wanted. Well, no, I couldn't play, really. But I found that if I turned up the automatic vibrato as fast as it would go, pushed in all the stops and played a lot of notes all together, it sounded like the Doors.

What I loved to do most, though, when I was alone in the church, was lie on my back in the sanctuary and watch the fans swoop around above. The beams and rafters were huge and black. I'm sure there hadn't been any direct sunlight up there since the day they'd put on the roof. It was a view I'd loved since I was five or six, when I'd lie on my mother's lap during the sermons and imagine I was climbing up there, swinging from the fan blades.

I'm still a daydreamer, now. I tell myself it's necessary,

that my mind is working on something important: file management, I suppose, or emotional issues my consciousness is still better off not knowing about. But none of that stops me from feeling guilty. I was raised a Presbyterian, the toughest sect in the entire Church of the Work Ethic. Even now I can see Mr. Donahue, the superintendent of the Sunday School, glaring down at me. "If your time isn't yours," he said, "it's somebody else's." I'm not sure what form of idleness I was indulging in at the time —perhaps only considering which one would be best— but he read me like a book.

Mr. Donahue would have disapproved mightily of my daydreaming away my extra time instead of working. That I was on the floor of the church would have been sloth most foul. But Mr. Donahue never caught me. Bob MacDonald did. I was on my back on the church floor with my head up, flying on the fans, when out of the corner of my eye I saw Bob and realized he must have been there a while.

I rarely saw Bob anywhere but on his way to work. He managed a series of apartment buildings, some of which he owned, and he always had three or four houses in various stages of renovation and repair. But he obviously still believed, at least theoretically, in the value of daydreaming. He laughed when I sat up, mussed my hair in his giant hands and took me to see the only two windows on the church that he didn't want me to paint.

They were tiny and intricate, and about forty feet off the ground, halfway up the steeple. Bob said he didn't want me up there by myself. He told me to leave them till the end and he would help.

So I finished the job and was paid, and, amazingly, I

found I'd made a profit. August went by, and September, too. Once in a while, on Sunday, I'd see Bob and ask him when we were going to paint the last two windows, but he never seemed too concerned. "That's the first thing to learn about a job," he told me. "It'll wait for you."

And it did. Right into November. It was snowing when he finally called. I wanted to show him all I'd learned, to let him watch me paint without making any mistakes, but it was Bob who went up the forty feet to the steeple, with me merely holding the ladder below. Still, it was fun to watch those huge hands at work again. He carefully cleaned the surface, dipped the brush deep into the can and slapped yellow paint all over the whole thing—sill, casement, glass and all. You couldn't even call it a window any more.

"That's the second thing to learn about a job," he said when he came back down. "Don't get fancy where nobody looks."

He was right. I was back at that church not long ago. Every bit of painting I did that summer has been long done over, except those two tiny windows. I guess nobody ever noticed. And Bob, in remarkably non-Presbyterian fashion, and probably having a lot of other things to do, never said a thing.

That's why I've been feeling a little more comfortable about taking it easy now and then, if no one's going to know the difference. I'm not planning on leaving the Church of the Work Ethic, I'm just thinking that maybe a Sunday off in the country isn't going to do any harm.

I like to think Bob MacDonald would have approved, and I hope he finally got to do a little of his own day-dreaming, too. He died, suddenly, a couple of years ago.

He wasn't very old. But, even by Presbyterian Work Ethic standards, he had done remarkably well. His kids were all married, he had eleven grandchildren, and he owned the biggest house in town. It had dozens of rooms, a pool, lots of extra space and was made of brick.

I don't remember a lot of wood showing on the outside of the place, so there wouldn't have been too much painting to keep up. What there was to do, well, I looked hard and I didn't see anything you'd have to get fancy over.

As to the rest, if Bob didn't get to it, I'm sure it'll wait.

Working the Room

I can vaguely remember laughing at older people for worrying about what the government did with their money. Now I am beginning to worry about what all those young ingrates are laughing about. It could be that complaining about the government is just part of the package once you've lived long enough to see how often it screws up. But, as I get older, I think the chief reason that old folks rant about taxes is for the entertainment. Complaining about the government is, no matter how ineffectual, something that seems to be more fun the longer you do it, and worrying about money, since it doesn't actually do anything about anything either, is a natural complement.

I had only just passed my thirty-fifth birthday when I found myself in one of the major centres of government-related money complaints: traffic court. And, oddly enough, I'd got there by trying to get out of paying for something.

The City of Toronto offers all kinds of educational programs for its children. They are mostly weekly courses, offered year-round, in a huge variety of disciplines, like swimming, ballet and karate, and most of them are absolutely free.

"The kindness of a socialist state," my neighbour said.

But space in these programs is limited. So, four or five times a year, otherwise normal and civilized Torontonians wake up long before the sun and stand in line to make sure their kids get a spot.

"The humiliation of a socialist state," my neighbour said.

If you live farther than walking distance from the sign-up place, you have to find somewhere to park. Of course, there are lots with parking metres only a few blocks away, and one could just spend a few more dollars that way, but, one morning not long ago, when I went to wait in line, I just happened to notice a spot on a residential street mere steps away.

It was a warm, spring morning. I got there early enough to get swimming lessons for one kid and Toddler Time for the other. Then, I walked back to the car and found a parking ticket on the windshield. It was a twenty-dollar fine for parking, without a permit, on a residential street between the hours of midnight and 8:00 a.m. My neighbour's car was parked nearby as well. He also had a ticket. In the interests of decency I'm not going to say what he said then, but, later on, he had a plan.

"If you dispute the ticket and sign up for French night court, the cop never shows and you don't have to pay," he said. Richard, my neighbour, is a Franco-Ontarian. He's as bilingual as a person can be. I'm as bilingual as *I* can be, which isn't the same thing at all. But if the cop wasn't going to show, I figured I'd be fine. Richard offered to sign me up, too.

The court date was a Thursday at 7:00 in the evening. We drove together, Richard and I, and paid for our parking.

There were a few cases on the docket before ours. I thought I'd just end up reading the copy of *Les Confessions* by Jean Jacques Rousseau that I'd brought along. But I didn't do much reading.

The judge was a woman in her mid-fifties, and this was her show. The way she blinked, if she yawned . . . everything hung on her. Or so it seemed.

First there was the case of the driver who was clocked at ninety kilometres per hour in a sixty zone. The cop who'd given her the ticket was there. He remembered seeing the red car flying down the street.

The driver maintained that he must have been mistaken. "It's impossible," she said. "I just don't drive that fast."

"But," the judge said, "we have both a radar report and an eyewitness that say you did."

The woman had nothing more to support her, but she still said it couldn't have happened, and that's when I felt another force in the court. I'll call it "the room." It was the way everyone else there responded to the story. They—we, I guess—were in this too. No one actually said anything about the speeder, but the room was giving its verdict loud and clear. She was lying. We knew. When the judge told her she had to pay, you could hear agreement exhaled from every direction.

The next case was a guy who ran a stop sign. We heard from the cop who'd caught him first. He was young, clean-cut and dressed in a suit. He spoke clearly, but with modesty. He looked exactly like what we all hoped a cop would be if we needed one. The room liked him right away.

The driver, on the other hand, was a loud and nasal-voiced man with an angular, mean-looking face and an attitude that said he resented being there and had plenty of more important things to be doing. It turned out he lived right beside the stop sign in question. It turned out he was a consulting engineer with an oil company. It turned out he drove a BMW.

The room bristled: a rich, obnoxious know-it-all who cared more about his Day-Timer than the safety of the neighbours' kids. He was going down.

The judge was tired of him, too, we could tell. But the driver wouldn't give in. He brought photographs of the intersection in question. He explained how he drove that street every day. He showed where the cop was parked, how long he'd been there, and how visible the cop car would have been.

"Look," he said, "how stupid would I have to be? I could see the policeman from down the block. He'd been there three days. Why would I roll through a stop sign in front of a cop who was put there to give out tickets for doing just that?" He looked at the judge. "Do *you* think I'm that stupid?"

There was what seemed like a very long pause. The engineer looked out at the room, and when it looked back, it seemed to have lost its conviction. I don't know if it was the judge or the room that swayed first, but the tide shifted very quickly. It was as if all of that emotion had simply been washed away in a single wave. In less than seconds, everyone had given the engineer the benefit of the doubt, and it seemed painfully obvious that he had been innocent all along. The judge agreed. He was off the hook.

Then they called Richard and me. It turned out that, because our officer had written two tickets on the same street and both drivers had asked for French night court, she'd shown up. It was show time.

Richard was first. He was courteous and articulate. He explained that these parking by-laws had been created to prevent people from leaving their cars overnight, not so they couldn't sign their kids up for programs. The judge agreed. And then it was my turn.

My French was a little stumbly, but all I really had to say was "I'm with him." When the judge asked what programs I was signing up for, I showed her the catalogue of choices.

It was quiet for a moment while she read. I looked around, and suddenly the question of whether the judge led the room, or vice versa, was crucial. The room, I could tell, had my number.

"Privileged Anglo-yuppie," it was saying. "Riding on free city programs, weaselling parking spots, and now pretending his first language is French when it clearly isn't, just so he can make us pay for luxuries he can well afford on his own!"

All true.

The silence was endless.

Then the judge looked at me over her glasses.

"*Qu'est-ce qu'ils font là, à* 'Toddler Time'*? Les chansons, les jeux?*" she asked. It turned out she had a niece in the neighbourhood. I almost thought she was going to ask me to sign her up next time! I got off.

I didn't stick around to try and figure out if the room would have swung my way, too. It seemed much harsher than our judge, in the end.

I suppose next time there's a sign-up day, I might just find out. That is, if the programs are still around. At this point, there seems to be some question about their survival in years to come. The City is saying we can't afford completely free programs any more. If that is the case, I guess I'll have to count myself lucky for learning as much about the judicial system as I did without going to jail. And even if the programs are cancelled, at least that will provide one more thing for me to complain about as I get older.

All part of living in a socialist state, I guess.

Premium Roulette

Okay, here's an idea. You give me money and I'll pay it back *if* you die.

All right, how about this? You give me money every month for a long time and if you have a terrible car accident I'll pay it back, but only if you *don't* die.

No, wait, I've got it. You give me money every month for a long time and I'll invest it. Then, if you die, I'll pay it back with interest, but not as much as I earned from it.

Okay, okay, this time for sure. You give me money in case you die, money in case you have a car accident and don't die, and more money in case you have a car accident and don't die but you kill somebody else, and a little more than that in case your house burns down, or you lose a limb, or you suffer some emotional trauma at work and can't earn money any more, and I'll keep all of that money and use it to hire good doctors and lawyers who will see things from my point of view, so, in case any of those things actually does happen to you, I won't have to pay back your money after all. Then I'll wear a suit, call myself one of the four pillars of finance and behave as if gambling on death and dismemberment is somehow respectable, and I'll be all set because even if you do endure something more awful than all of the possibilities listed above, I'll call it an Act of God, which won't be covered in our agreement, which I'll call a policy.

You wouldn't think we were talking about a sound business plan, would you?

Well, apparently, it is. It is difficult to get precise figures, I've found, on just how much money is tied up in insurance of one kind or another at any time, but it is safe to say that the numbers easily run into the trillions. It is a mind-numbingly huge and profitable industry, and it does indeed regard itself as one of the four pillars of finance. Mind you, the other three are "Give me your money and I'll charge you to use it" (banks), "Give me your money and I'll pretend it's more important to me than mine is" (trust companies) and "Make me a partner in your company and I'll walk away when you're in trouble" (brokerage houses).

Insurance fits right in.

But the real reason insurance is so successful, and so odious, has to do with how it looks at people. Insurance looks at people the only way it can and still stay in business: it doesn't. It looks at *groups* of people, along with groups of diseases, groups of accidents, groups of crimes, groups of natural disasters . . . the more the better.

The earliest recorded insurance contracts go back to the Babylonian Empire. There's no reason to believe that the notion of betting money on disaster wasn't around long before that, but Babylonia in 3000 to 4000 BC was ripe for the invention of insurance. It had the two main ingredients in spades. First of all, the Babylonians were pioneers in complex mathematics, and Babylon, the capital city, was a major port. Every year, great numbers of ships sailed in and out of the port, and, every year, an increasingly predictable number of them ended up sinking. Math and disaster—bingo! All Bobby Babylon had to do was sit on the banks of the Tigris or the Euphrates and keep track of the sinkers and swimmers, and he could go into the bottomry business.

That's what they called it back then, a bottomry contract, but whether that name has anything to do with where the ships at the losing end of the deal ended up, I don't know. A bottomry contract was a fairly simple affair. Merchants borrowed money at very high rates, sometimes 25 or 30 percent, to finance a given shipment of goods, with the boat as collateral. If all went well, the loan was repaid when the boat returned to port. If the boat went down, the loan was forgiven.

Bobby Babylon's Bottomry: We Bet Big Bucks Your Boat Gets Back.

Business boomed.

The key was in the numbers. If Bobby could step back and simply look at the averages, and if traffic along the Euphrates was high enough to give him a decent sample size for his calculations, his predictions were bound to keep him above water. But if Bobby's customers wanted to borrow money against more diversified Babylonian interests—say, the building of giant towers in the centre of town—all bets were off. As long as the numbers were high, charting the comings and goings of ships and typhoons worked fine for Bobby and his lentil-counters in the claims department.

This system of marine insurance stayed much the same for the next 5,600 years, when a man named Edward Lloyd began listing shipping information under the soup du jour in his seventeenth-century London dockyard coffee house. This made him popular with merchants, bankers and insurance underwriters. It doubtless took its toll on the place's ambiance, but it did produce results. Edward Lloyd's table d'hôte eventually gave birth to the publication known as Lloyd's List, and the enormously powerful Lloyd's of London, which still exists today. The ambiance in the business is still a little dry, but that's okay. Lloyd's, and the industry that evolved from those gents who sat around the bar chatting easily about vast loss of life and shocking personal tragedy, doesn't actually deal with the public any more.

That left an opening, though, and before too long, someone with a little more interpersonal skill and even less conscience stumbled into the coffee house, or the boardroom, and realized that perhaps the most valuable cargo on those ships wasn't the dry goods that might end up as wet goods, or even the blocks and mortar for the building of very tall towers. No. The real cash cargo on those boats wasn't in the hold but in the bunks. It was the crew members, especially if they had families who'd be upset, or at least financially put out, when Johnny didn't come sailing home.

Life insurance first turned up in ancient Rome, where there were burial societies that collected monthly dues against eventual funeral costs. But it really took off centuries later, in a huge, wealthy, young and naive land full of people who behaved like a school of fish and thought of themselves as individuals. America loved life insurance—an idea that purported to view each person as an individual and treated them all like a school of fish.

The first life insurance company in the American

colonies was the Presbyterian Ministers' Fund, organized in 1759. I'm not making this up. Now, although the Presbyterians are no longer directly involved, they certainly left their mark. As of 1990, $9.4 trillion was tied up in life insurance in the United States. Now there's an Act of God!

Life insurance wasn't the only branch of the business to start fishing for clients between shipwrecks. It was just the first. Now there's homeowner's insurance, car insurance, disability insurance and many others, and they all work on the same principle. They treat their customers, and their tragedies, as a group, but sell to them one at a time. At least that, so to speak, is the claim. It's just a little bit difficult to process. Monoliths, especially ones that think of a human life as a mildly interesting numeric pattern, are not particularly welcome when they come knocking at the door.

Enter the insurance broker.

The broker, the carefully constructed image tells us, is not a giant, unfeeling corporation. He or she is a free agent, lobbying the monoliths on our behalf. He or she is a caring person, whose only goal in life (and in long-term disability) is to protectively wrap loving and sympathetic arms around the customer in times of need—even the poor sod who's been run over by a garbage truck or lost his wife or had his riverside dream home washed away by a monstrous wave following the collapse of a downtown tower into the Euphrates.

But that image of the caring broker is simply porthole dressing. He or she can hug us till the ships come home but will rarely be able to give us any money for our trouble. The insurer does that, and once we are placed within *those* loving arms, we cease to be a pathetic, garbage-trampled, homeless, slightly dampened widower and become claim number 25,678,443.B: a potential liability, however negligible, to be disputed tooth and nail, and the justification for any number of arbitrary and stupefying rate increases.

This is love and sympathy?

Not that I'd actually *want* to be hugged by my broker. There is something, I think, about a line of work that cheerfully examines each of the most horrific potential calamities in a life that would take the humanity out of even the most beguiling personality.

"Perils?" I remember asking Sam, my first broker, after he'd listed the terms of our agreement. That's what the insurance industry calls any of the terrible things that could happen to you, a "peril." It makes no difference to them whether it's a sliver in your foot or a cleaver through your neck, it's a peril. The other word they like is "loss," which could mean a bicycle or a life. Life, according to Sam, is full of perils, some of which result in loss. In my case, the loss was a bicycle.

But my loss hadn't been caused by anything particularly perilous. I'd simply come all the way downtown in a hurry before I noticed I'd left my lock at home. I was meeting a colleague in a big office tower and my bike had to stay outside. It was a beautiful bike, too. More expensive than any I'll ever own again, I'm sure. Light as air and as fast as the wind. It was sure to be stolen in minutes.

Then, across the street, I saw salvation. A building I knew well. People inside I could trust. It was a Presbyterian church.

I never saw the bike again.

But that's not fair. The church sexton *did* watch it for me, for a while, but he had things to do. I took too long getting back. The bike was parked in a little passageway that was as far as I could get from any of the main doors, but, like all churches, this was a public building, and a busy downtown one at that. Anyone could have taken it. I can really only blame myself. Still, I can't help thinking that if it had been 1759, I might have at least been able to buy a policy in the church office before I went from peril to loss. As it was, it was 1988, and I went from riding the wind, to walking the sidewalk, to a pay phone, to calling Sam.

"Perils," he said. "You've got your 'Named Perils,' which would include your fire, your lightning, your theft, your explosions and windstorms..."

"On a bike?" I asked.

". . . but you wouldn't be covered for your freezing, your water leakage, your termite damage, your rust, your mould, your dry rot, your contamination, your smog, your settling and cracking, your loss from animals or insects, or from earth movement, your flood, your war, your spoilage or neglect, which are your Acts of God."

"It *was* stolen from a church," I said.

"Of course some perils are your named perils but are not the only cause of loss. If you're covered for fire but after your fire there's a landslide or a flood or..."

I hung up and walked home. My house was still standing. And I did buy homeowner's insurance, eventually. It wasn't pleasant, and it wasn't cheap, but still, the next time loss came my way, I was ready, right?

Wrong.

Two years ago someone stole our double stroller. I'm

still not sure what to make of this. The stroller was an in-line model, rather than the trendier side-by-side. It was far from new-looking and had some nasty steering problems with anything close to a full load. Still, it, along with our wagon (which had steering problems of its own), was stolen off our front porch in the middle of a bright and sunny afternoon. I've spent some time since on the board-walk looking for a family listing to starboard, but so far, nothing has turned up.

Anyway, neither did my insurance. The real peril, it turned out, wasn't the thief, who, if you think about it, had already stooped low enough to be far more pathetic than perilous. The real peril was the deductible.

The deductible, if you haven't had the pleasure, is the amount above which your insurer will compensate you for any given loss. So, if you have in your basement an antique soap-box derby car made of teak and mahogany, designed by Frank Lloyd Wright, and it is stolen, resulting in a claim of $20,000, if your deductible is $100, the insurer will pay you $19,900. All very reasonable.

But you don't, I'm willing to bet, have a $20,000 soap-box derby car in your basement. You might, on the other hand, have a double stroller on your front porch.

So, when your neighbourhood is beset one spring by a rash of double stroller thefts,[1] the kind folks in your

[1] This really happened. The police officer I talked with said it happens every spring. Double strollers are expensive, not widely available, and easy to steal. This is because in any dwelling with two or more small children, whatever parent or guardian may be present is far too exhausted to even think of guarding the front porch, let alone chasing after a fleeing felon in a speeding stroller, no matter what kind of steering problems it has.

insurer's actuarial department spend the summer figuring out how much it cost them to replace each double stroller, which, let's say, turns out to be $300. Then, sometime in the fall, with, after all, plenty of time before the stroller-stealing season starts up again, they quietly inform you by way of tiny little notes[2] on your statement that your deductible has now been raised to $500 (just in case someone in your neighbourhood *does* have a Frank Lloyd Wright soap-box derby car and has left *it* out on the porch, too), and that if you want to maintain your $100 deductible your insurance will now cost vast amounts more.

This means that when your double stroller—and, just to be cruel, your wagon—are stolen on that fine spring day, and you call your agent to find out if you are covered, they can say that yes, you are, but it's probably going to be under your deductible.

Peril. Loss. You can see why they use these words.

At the time of writing, I've just returned from my weekly basketball game, and, as a thirty-seven-year-old white male, exactly halfway through my life expectancy, at this point my chief named perils are fatigue, sore feet and an inconsistent jump shot.

And, coincidentally, my yearly life insurance bill arrived in the mail today. I'm sure they'd be happy to know I'm exercising. Not because they want me to live to a ripe and happy old age—they don't care about that. I've got term life insurance. They sold me a policy based on the perils I posed at the time of signing, and the chances of my incurring a loss during the term of my coverage, which, in my

---

[2] About this big.

case, is until I turn thirty-nine. At this point, their only concern is that I stay healthy enough to make it to thirty-nine years, zero days, zero hours and one second. After that, my policy expires, and so can I, as far as they are concerned. As long as they're rid of the peril of paying up, whether I hop companies or hop the twig is no longer of any consequence. Or, if I stay with the world, and them, to launch into another nine-year segment of living, they'll send a friendly nurse around to my place to listen to my heart and ask questions about my stress levels and my work and my marriage and my children, the kinds of things a concerned friend asks about. Then, on the basis of that report, they'll gouge me for even higher premiums.

Personally, I haven't felt the least bit risky, to anyone, in about ten years, which is about when I started buying insurance.

Incidentally, when I first called Sam ten years ago, he did use the phrase "Act of God." I've since learned it's been replaced by "Catastrophic Loss." I think that's too bad. I kind of liked the idea of God causing a little trouble now and then. As inexplicable as His motives might be for releasing a flood, or stirring up a little political insurrection, or even turning a blind eye to a front porch stroller theft, at least if there's some order behind the horror, there might be some behind the joy, too.

But I suspect insurance had less philosophical reasons for replacing Him as their chief suspect in the perpetration of unpredictable perils and losses. I think they didn't like the competition. They're getting awfully big and God-like themselves. And it's not just insurance. The banks are buying into the business, too. So are the trust companies. And everybody's buying the brokerage houses.

As if that weren't enough, they keep announcing mergers. Pretty soon it won't matter which bank or insurance company you go to, they'll all be the same one, with the same high rates and ridiculous policies and deductibles that go up faster than you can steal a bike from a church.

It's not that I mourn the loss of the small, independent financial services provider. I'm not sure he, she or it ever existed to begin with. It's just that, as pompous as it sounded, I think that "four pillars of finance" thing might not have been a bad idea. It's a good building plan, four pillars. You could make an awfully big tower that way. But once you start combining pillars, and building higher and higher, and it begins to look like you might not stop until you reach the sky, well, it's a lot harder to know exactly what might happen under those circumstances.

Any bets?

Bodily Harmony

I figure a person's relationship with his or her body passes through three distinct phases over the course of a life.

The first is the "Stranger" phase. As infants, I'm told, we have no concept where our own bodily boundaries end and our mother's begin. We have no say in what our body does. We have no idea why it does any of those things, how we might get it to stop or why, particularly, when it does one or two of them, our parents begin to mutter under their breath and argue over whose turn it is this time.

Into childhood and adolescence, the body becomes more understood and familiar, but it is still full of surprises. "Hey!" the four-year-old cries when she finds she is spending more time on her ice skates than on her bum. "Hey!" the twelve-year-old cries when he finds an eruption on his nose. "Hey!" the fourteen-year-old girl says to herself in the pool change room when her bathing suit top finally begins to fit.

By early adulthood, though, person and body have a great thing going. This is the glorious "Teflon" stage. The mid-twenty-year-old can do anything to his or her body: heat it, shake it, stir it and bake it well beyond any normally advisable temperature for days on end, and then throw it in the sink and forget about it, and it still bears no permanent mark.

The trouble is, the only indication that the body won't always be able to withstand that kind of treatment without considering it abuse is that, all of a sudden, it *is* abuse.

This is the beginning of the final phase of the person/body relationship. I call it the "Retrospective" stage, because with each incremental lapse into decrepitude, we are forced to account for the many wondrous qualities we will now have to do without. The Retrospective phase is full of discoveries: how wonderfully supple the body once was, how brutally stiff it can be now, how much more so in years to come, how many things can go wrong all at once to make it that way, and how little the medical profession understands any of it.

That is not to say that our lives from thirty on are unrelenting misery. On the contrary, it is only in the post-thirty years that a person is free to concentrate on other things. Surprise pimples are rarer, and so is the urge to stay up all night dancing and heaving and, well, okay, the lack of urge may be cause for some worry, but still—the body, until the final years, anyway, ceases to be the focus of obsession.

For most of the Retrospective stage, the body is simply a vehicle. And travelling in an old, familiar vehicle can be nice at times. Older vehicles have bigger trunks. The seat is worn just the way you like it. It's relaxing. You can whistle along with the bumps and ticks of the internal radio and know which noises are worth pulling over for and which can be ignored without risk of a breakdown.

And if you have to pull into the right lane more than you'd like, so the twenty-something speed demons can flail by, leaning on the horn, you can feel sure their day will come. You might even pass them in a few years. If not, you can take comfort in the bumper sticker that best sums up the long, slow, downhill ride into the last half of the journey of life: "Don't Laugh," it says. "It's Paid For."

Bound and Clogged

I have a vivid memory of a lunch I enjoyed with a good friend a few years ago. It was just before Christmas. The ridiculous rush of extra work that has to be done was almost over, and the inevitable exhaustion that ruins the holiday hadn't quite set in.

We went to a restaurant specializing in the provision of large quantities of very rich and decadent food. We spread the foie gras thick as mortar on bricks of crusty bread. We broke the lobster shells with our hands. We laughed and we drank and it was wonderful. In my mind, I can still taste it. Which, one day, might have to be enough. Soon after that lunch I learned that those foods were taking a toll on more than just my wallet, and, if I kept eating them, I'd end up with the kind of bill that would be paid in full only when I cashed out, myself. The problem was that my cholesterol was high.

Actually, it was quite high. At least my doctor thought it was. She had to do some more tests. But, in the meantime, just to be safe, I gave up foie gras and did some research.

What I learned is that there is more than one kind of cholesterol. There *is* such a thing as good cholesterol. It's big and heavy and sweeps out the corners, like a Zamboni of the arteries. The trouble is, as with most things, most people end up with some bad along with the good. And the bad *is* bad. It hangs around your bloodstream like hoods at a convenience store. One day you go in for a cream puff, take a bite and *wham*! it jumps your ticker, and before you know it, you haven't just bought the cream puff, you've bought the farm.

There isn't a whole lot of concise and definitive information on the topic of good cholesterol (a.k.a. High Density Lipoproteins, HDL, Zamboni of the arteries) or bad cholesterol (a.k.a. Low Density Lipoproteins, LDL, venal and arterial convenience store hoods). Nobody seems to be too sure about any of this. The experts link the bad cholesterol to heart disease, but they still can't say for certain that it is a cause. Some people live to be ninety-nine with the stuff piled up in their blood like snowbanks in Thunder Bay.

I'd like to think I'm one of them. I'm almost assuming I am. As it turns out, the greater portion of my high cholesterol is HDL, the good kind. So, it's really almost something I don't need to think about any more. Well, not much. The trouble is, if I do need to think about it, I won't find out until it's a little late in the game.

Until then, the experts have plenty of suggestions on how I might best cope with the situation. Yes, these are the same experts who aren't sure it really is a problem. Somehow they are much more certain about treatment. They say, from their own cushy positions, that I could exercise vigorously for forty minutes a day, five days a week, for an entire year and check it again. Chances are it will have all cleared up.

Or not.

Others say I can drink alcohol in moderation, one drink per day. Far preferable, in terms of treatment, really. And some of the experts are convinced it works. *They* think the reason people have high cholesterol isn't because of their lack of activity but because of their abundance of stress. One drink a day serves to loosen up the individual and his bloodstream, too. That way I can relax, stop thinking so much about my cardiac health, watch a little hockey, play canasta and coast into old age without another thought.

Or not.

I could move to France. That one's got the experts really stumped. The French aren't famous for holding back where food, or anything else, is concerned (except perhaps compliments for non-French people). But as a nation they have a remarkably low rate of heart disease. As explanations go, the experts are about as definite on this one as any other, but most suggest that the health of the French heart is a result of attitude. The French drink wine. They eat long, slow meals and blow up islands in the South Pacific only after a good, long afternoon nap.

The other thing I can do, of course, is change my diet. That's the one that I found myself thinking of the most.

The phone rang just as I was sitting down to a piece of mincemeat pie. My mother's. It was left over from Christmas. I'd only had one bite. It was the receptionist from the doctor's office calling. All she said was "Your cholesterol is high," but those four words changed everything. When I came back to the table, that pie, that wonderful pie, was no longer reminding me of cherished childhood Christmases, it was trying to kill me.

I found myself daydreaming about the dark food flings of my youth.

Bodily Harmony

I worked for a while at a Russian restaurant in New York. I worked the cold station, which meant making the salads and the cold plates and some desserts, stocking the smoked fish and the goose breast and the quails' eggs and the caviar. Lots of caviar, actually: Sevruga, Osetrova, Beluga—all of which I knew nothing about. But I made it my business to learn. I sampled it often to discern the subtleties of flavour and texture. So often, in fact, that after a few days a colleague took me aside and told me how much the stuff cost. By then, I was surprised to learn, I'd already consumed more than I could replace with a week's salary.

I didn't tell the owner. He had enough to worry about.

The place was brand new. He was hoping it would become the favourite haunt of a very small and very wealthy Upper East Side clientele. Consequently, everything had to be absolutely fresh and stocked in abundance. The chosen few could arrive any day, and they wouldn't want to wait.

But the very wealthy don't hurry many places, and the weeks dragged on, often with no one in the place but the lowly labourers and their nervous employer. We opened only for lunch and dinner, so mornings found the fridges and counters and pantries full to overflowing with the previous night's fabulous riches, already slightly too old for the fabulously rich. There were pastries—napoleons and apple tarts and croissants. The bartender had a way with a twelve-hour-old Blue Mountain blend that made a cup of mud to straighten your tie. And the sous-chef, Bill, developed a specialty that I have yet to experience anywhere else. It was a paper-thin omelette stuffed with fragrant, butter-sautéed mushrooms and white pepper, gently coated in a white truffle Hollandaise.

Beyond breakfast, though, the daily routine was a considerable letdown. The kitchen fan broke on opening day. No one bothered to fix it, and by mid-morning most days the kitchen was a sauna. My work station had been built so close to the swinging dining-room doors that a waiter in a hurry (and there isn't any other kind) could give me a concussion. There were no reliable recipes. The menu changed every day, and the chef, the only person who knew that menu, often slept right through lunch and showed up mid-afternoon.

On top of all of that, I had lied my way into the job in the first place, hoping to learn on the fly. I was in completely over my head. The chef knew it but was too tired to help. Bill knew it, but he was too busy saving his own job. And, worst of all, Carlos, the Dominican dishwasher, who called me Jimmy, no matter how much I corrected him, knew it better than anyone and took great delight in cheering as I flailed my way through shift after disastrous shift. "Jimmy!" he'd call as the chef bellowed for a mousse he'd needed fifteen minutes ago. "Jimmy! You fucked up! Go, Jimmy, go! Ha! Ha!"

When, inevitably, I was fired, I wasn't particularly happy. But the owner took me aside. He told me I had to learn when it was time to step aside and move on. This was the man who, every night, strolled among the tables with a guitar, singing all fourteen verses of "The Volga Boatman." But still, he was right.

Everyone watched as I walked downstairs to my locker, packed up my fat-soaked clothes and shoes and came back out, through the silent kitchen, into the street, without my last day's pay. The last thing I heard was Carlos calling

"Bye, bye, Jimmy!" and the owner yelling at everyone to get back to work.

I don't often think about those things when I remember the Russian restaurant, though. I think of the breakfasts. They made all of that worthwhile, and more. I don't think of the week, month or, *ulp*, years that job might have taken off my final quota of time on the planet. It's still hard to regret those mornings. Even when I found my cholesterol levels were about to laugh at me and call me Jimmy, as far as I was concerned, it would still be better to have chowed and croaked than never to have chowed at all.

Then I went for further tests.

My doctor sent me to a nutritionist. She had me write down everything I ate for a week. It wasn't as horrific a display as I had feared, but there were some things that just had to go. Cheese was out. Butter was out. Dough with lots of cheese and butter was *really* out.

That was a problem. At this point I'm quite willing to admit that I am a doughboy, and I always will be. Some people, when life sets in and won't back off, console themselves with a bucket of Häagen-Dazs and a spoon. Others reach for noodles, or mashed potatoes, or their credit cards, and still others, I'm told, reach for a rubber suit and a cat-o'-nine-tails. Fair enough. I'm in no position to judge. I am a fool for dough. Rich, gooey, only-good-for-a-few-minutes-after-it's-out-of-the-oven-and-never-worth-the-calories-it-takes-to-get-through-the-crust dough. Doughnuts, croissants, cinnamon rolls, strudel, honeybuns—the lot.

Now, according to my nutritionist, all of that was gone

for me. One look at my chart and the dough in my life fell like a cake in a thunderstorm. My dough intake was not just to be reduced, it was to be eradicated for three whole months, to see if my cholesterol levels would come back into line.

It was hard to know which side to cheer for. If my numbers didn't get any lower with all of that fat reduction, I wouldn't have to think about my diet again. I was probably going to have a heart attack at a very young age and die. On the other hand, if my cholesterol levels *did* relate to my diet, I could control them—by eating cardboard and grass clippings and crossing the street at the smell of a bakery for the rest of my miserable days.

Or not. Right? I was hanging on to that: the blissful ignorance option. I've complained about doctors being a lot more in the dark than they let on, but this time they were on my side. Go indecision! Go denial! Say you can't be sure! Bring up the old "quality of life" argument!

That last one, I discovered, was worth cheering about. By the early 1990s, cholesterol really *was* ruining quality of life. Not because of overall health, but because of overwhelming hype. If cholesterol wasn't inescapable, endless talk about it was. It was on every talk show, every magazine cover—and in the Ice Man, too! Remember him—the intrepid Alps traveller from 3300 BC who was found largely intact, and frozen solid? Doctors performed an autopsy and found his arteries were as hard as peanut brittle. "Cholesterol killed Ice Man!" headlines screamed. That he was estimated to be something over five thousand years old at the time was deemed a secondary health concern.

I even saw "no cholesterol" stickers on a bin of bananas. This is like putting a notice on a pencil case to alert the unwary that it does not contain a hockey stick. At the same time, potato chip manufacturers began to boast that their products didn't contain cholesterol either. This is true, chips do not contain cholesterol. People do. They may as well have said that chips won't make you fat. That's true too, as long as you don't eat them.

I happen to be acquainted with a rather prominent expert in the field of hypertension and cardiac health. His name is Dr. Alexander Logan. As cholesterol labels spread their gooey way into the banana market, and into the consciousness of the general public, he began to wonder not so much about the effect of the goo as about the effect of the label.

He told me about studies involving the popular health world's previous *maladie-du-jour*: high blood pressure. Researchers knew high blood pressure was a very serious health risk, but almost worse, they found, was being told about it. The results were shocking. Once they'd been told their blood pressure was a problem and that they should do something about it, people's marriages got rocky. Their careers stalled. They were less successful in almost every area of life than their non-labelled counterparts, and worse, they just weren't as happy, even after they'd corrected the problem. The label did permanent damage.

Dr. Logan wanted to know what effect a high-cholesterol label would have.

So did I.

I'd been wearing my label for about six months when I talked to him. I hadn't noticed myself being particularly less happy, but, it was true I hadn't been given a promotion at work and my wife was getting awfully mad at me. Especially for buying all those bananas.

Dr. Logan found, strangely enough, that being told about your high cholesterol didn't do any of those bad things to your life. He found that people who knew about their high cholesterol had just as many promotions as they would have had otherwise, just as much fun, and, if they stopped buying bananas, their marriages worked out as well, or as poorly, as they would have anyway.

What surprised him, though, was that he also found that people with high cholesterol were actually much happier than those without. Not happier with their health, necessarily (or their jobs and marriages and shopping habits), just happier, period. What they found so cheering about the cheese piled up in the corners of their bloodstream, planning to kill them prematurely, he couldn't say. But there you have it.

Hearing all that made me even happier. My friend and I celebrated with another decadent lunch. It's true. I also went back to a lot of my old eating habits and basically stopped thinking about my diet. I broke all my appointments with the nutritionist and never called her back. I haven't gone back to my doctor to have my levels checked in three years.

So, it's not true that you can't go back home to dough and blissful ignorance. It's just a long trip, you need a good boat, and you have to travel by the darkest emotional waterway there is: denial.

At least there's lots of good company—all those happy-go-lucky folks with their veins all bound and clogged, all wondering about moving to France. I don't know what the statistics are for happy-in-the-face-of-relatively-certain-death former bass trombonist radio hosts who go there in their late thirties, but how bad could they be?

Besides, I'm going to be taking that longer, final journey at some point anyway, right? And I can't say I know what's coming after that, but the way I see it, whatever it is, it'll be a lot nicer on a full stomach.

Beat the Clock

Before any further discussion of aging, how about a step back to look at the chief agent of bodily deterioration? Time, and the enjoyment of its passage, is both a guarantee of happiness and a reminder of the certainty of death. With power like that, you'd hope it would have a system to its madness, or, at least, as most guarantees do, carry with it a clearly set out list of rules and limitations.

I began to wonder about those rules and limitations one afternoon last December, as I was going home from work. When I stepped out of the subway that night, I couldn't help noticing that it was pitch black outside. Absolutely middle-of-the-night dark. I wasn't even home yet, let alone sitting in my favourite chair and enjoying the fine feeling of accomplishment that sweeps a person up at the end of a working day and fills him with a deep sense of warmth as his wonderful partner-in-life listens intently to his moving insights and his full-of-character yet obedient children put themselves to bed quietly, efficiently and all by themselves.

None of that had happened yet. But that was not my problem. My problem was that it wasn't nighttime yet. It wasn't even dinnertime.

Why do we pretend our days are the same length all year round, when every other living being on the planet knows they aren't? We're diurnal. Diurnal animals do their survival business during the day, and at night they sit in their favourite chairs and enjoy fine feelings of accomplishment. At least, I assume they do. I don't see the other members of the diurnal mammalian community coming home to the den or the warren or the hutch in the dead-of-night darkness. Why do I have to stay working long after the sun has packed it in, just because the little hand isn't yet on the five? Should I really follow a ten-dollar watch in preference to something as vast and powerful as the Sun?

Why not, I wondered, calculate the passage of the hours based on the amount of available sunlight? If we have decided we need twenty-four hours in every day, fine, but why does one hour always have to be as long as the other? It's not as if the passage of time is uniform in any other part of life. Those evenings of quiet reflection, I'm told, if they ever do come around, are so delightful that they are over in a flash. On the other hand, I know from personal experience that if you are on the radio, and you have nothing to say, forty-five seconds can be as long as three hours.

So, given that, in our temperate climate, all else is variable from one season to another, why not allow for variable hours? It might not be too bad. In December, for example, in most parts of Canada, the daylight hours would only last about forty minutes, but who wouldn't want to work shorter hours? Time already vanishes inexplicably at work. This way we'd be facing up to it.

And who is to say that even those daylight hours should be all the same length? The first three hours of the working day are the only time anybody gets anything done. Let's make them, say, ninety minutes each, more or less, with another ninety for lunch, so we can finish our pudding, with the remaining hours as short as we'd like them to be that day, as long as they're all finished by sundown.

The evenings would be fabulous. There would be time to put the kids to bed, do the dishes, sweep the floor, vacuum the car, clean the cat box, call a few friends and read the paper all in the space of an hour. That is, the hour immediately after dinner, which could be at least two hours long and still leave plenty of time for the other fifteen we'd need to fit in before sunrise, with the option of a few short ones in the middle of the night, so that lying awake from three to four wouldn't be so depressing.

Of course, come June, we'd all be working almost all the time—but who watches the hockey playoffs these days, anyway?

I was feeling pretty good about this little system, when I found I'd missed discovering it by something like two thousand years. Way back then, when the world was an agricultural, pre-industrial society, we had only one big timepiece, the Sun, and everybody lived according to its dictates without considering otherwise. They really did live a working day like the one I've just described.

It was Bert Hall who broke my bubble. He's an associate professor at the University of Toronto. He told me that the notion of coordinated, universal time is relatively new—and that, in some ways, it doesn't actually work. Time zones, for example, can be a problem.

I know they're a good Canadian invention, and that if it weren't for Sir Sandford Fleming trains would have to spend so much time fixing their clocks they'd never get anywhere—let alone get anywhere on time, whatever that means. But still, we've evolved a system where it's the same time in Bath, Maine, as it is in Wawa, Ontario. How can that be? Those two cities are more than two days' drive apart, at any time of year. When bath time is over according to Bath time, the sun is at its lowest and the kids pull the plug. Meanwhile, in northern Ontario, a lot of Wawa is still in the tub. It's ridiculous.

Solar time would solve all of that. The whole thing is arbitrary, anyway, and since we've already deregulated everything else in Canada, why not time? Besides, in many ways, it's already happened. The city of Toronto has had its own time system for years.

If you ask a native Torontonian how long it will take to get from where you are to just about anywhere else in the city, the answer will always be the same: "About forty-five minutes." This is not true. You can't get anywhere in Toronto in forty-five minutes. It takes an hour to get to the corner store for a Popsicle. I'm not talking about any dark-of-winter relative-duration hours, either. These are real, sixty-minute hours.

It's not that Torontonians are uniformly deceptive or unfriendly to outsiders. Well, not much . . . but that is not the point. Everyone who has lived here longer than a little while (and I can't be any more specific about exactly how long *a little while* is . . .) knows how long things will take. "Forty-five minutes," in Toronto, really means something like "About as long as you would expect it to take." It's the locally accepted unit of time.

And I think that's fine. Time *is* different here. This is a city that worships a hockey team that hasn't won in thirty years, no matter how late the playoffs run.

Anyway, Toronto is not alone in this. Every place has its own temporal vernacular.

A friend of mine has a farm near Chesley, Ontario. She says that, for her and her husband, the largest unit of local time is a trip to town, as in "That'd take you about a trip to town." A smaller unit is a conversation with a neighbour, and the smallest division of the daylight passage of time might be a walk down the lane to get the mail. It's how she divides her day. Naturally, there are irregularities. This same couple measures the start of the day by the unit of "one shower." The trouble is, if it's her shower, he has enough time to make a cup of coffee. If it's his, she may as well start making dinner.

Napoleon was perhaps the first to redefine time for more than just his own purposes. He thought, as a lot of people have, that the months should really be all the same length, 30 days. That meant, if you had twelve of them, you'd have 360 days in the year, which was just right, the same as the degrees in a circle.

Except that a year, one trip around the Sun, doesn't take 360 days. It takes 365. "*Eh, bien*!" Napoleon said. "So what? We'll guillotine the year where we want and have a five-day party afterward!"

They did, too, and once they'd cleaned up, they started the year again at Day One. If the Emperor hadn't been so keen on shoving the idea down the throats of all the other time zones in Europe, we might still be using that system today. Our current one is certainly no more accurate. It's not that we haven't learned anything since Napoleon. We just haven't changed. And since there's no hurry—it's June, now, plenty of daylight left—let's back up a bit.

At first, people thought the Earth took 365 of its own

rotations (days) to orbit the Sun (one year). Then, sometime around the year 300 BC, scientists (they were keeners on this stuff back then) found it actually took the Earth 365.25 days to go around the Sun—about six hours longer than one year. So, scientists of the day invented the leap year. Every four years, they added one day, and presto! We were all set.

Until about 1500.

Somewhere around then, Christian authorities began to get nervous. They had fixed the date of Easter, the celebration of the resurrection of Christ, that which separated them from all the other churches, so that it fell exactly on March 21 on the Julian calendar, every year. That day, they said, at sunrise, was the precise moment at which the body of Christ had risen from the tomb and ascended into the Kingdom of Heaven.

But something was wrong. Even if the Son of God's timetable had been accurate, the Church's wasn't. Astronomers had long suspected something was slipping because, although the days were clicking by exactly as they were supposed to, it just didn't seem quite as chilly on the toes in the sandals at the sunrise service as it used to.

It was Christopher Clavius who finally set things straight. He was an adviser to Pope Gregory XIII, and he figured out that the Earth wasn't taking 365.25 days to go around the Sun, it was taking 365.2425 days. That might not sound like a big difference, but by 1582 it meant the entire calendar was off by two weeks. Two weeks! Christ wasn't just rising on Easter morning, he was long gone and happily sitting on the right hand of God enjoying the view, and the folks down below hadn't even begun to warm up the pump organ.

So, in 1582, on the advice of Clavius, Pope Gregory XIII set things right. He said good night to his subjects on Thursday, October 4 at midnight, and when they woke up the next day, it was Friday, October 19.

Now, from a temporal management point of view, this was heads-up thinking, and even over four hundred years later there's no one to challenge him as Time's Man of the Year in 1582. But that was probably small comfort for the rest of the folks, especially the farm worker who was told he'd just lost two weeks' wages because of a clerical error in the Vatican. Faith in the Church was tested on many levels that night, and a lot of people's patience wound up about two weeks too short.

Things are easier now. These years, to avoid the two-week cutaway, the calendar experts make sure we skip a leap year every four hundred years. That is, every fourth turn-of-the-century year, like the one that is coming up, is not a leap year. If you're upset about losing that day at the end of February, talk to the Pope. It's nothing to do with me.

Keeping track of time sure can get messy. And that's just the story on the length of the year as one, large unit. When you start to look into how to divide *that* up, things get worse by the, er, moment.

The business of months has all kinds of vagaries attached to it. There's the Julian calendar and the Gregorian calendar and the Lunar calendar and none of them is actually based on anything that holds up scientifically any more. But we have to live by something, and having twelve months works about as well as anything else. Twelves are neat. You can cut them up a whole bunch of ways, and, from a management point of view, twelves come in handy, whether you're into digits or disciples. There aren't too many other numbers that can say that. Threes are big, but twelves have four of them, and a couple of sixes, too. Still, beyond lots of high-end hooey that isn't of any use to a disgruntled farm worker wondering where his paycheque went, the number of months could have been any number, really. The same is true for the number of hours, or minutes, or seconds. The whole thing is just what somebody came up with ages ago to get us through the night.

And the most shocking realization for me was that the same is true for the week. The Judaic calendar was calculated on the lunar cycle. That is, it takes twenty-eight days for the Moon to circle the Earth—a number easily divisible by seven. Also, at the time, they knew of only seven planets, so they named one day for each planet and had four seven-day weeks.[1]

Don't get me wrong, I like the week. I like Sunday mornings. I like Monday nights. Thursday is long but it's closer to Saturday. To me, the week is real. It's my life. But we now know a lunar cycle isn't exactly twenty-eight days. It's actually closer to thirty. So we might just as easily decide to have two fifteen-day weeks, three of ten, or worse, five six-day weeks, or six of five days each.

What would I do with my weekends? Which day would be garbage day? Would there still be Bay Days? What

---

[1] After Sunday, think of the French: *lundi* (Moon Day), *mardi* (Mars Day), *mercredi* (Mercury Day), *jeudi* (Jupiter Day), *vendredi* (Venus Day) and *samedi* (Saturn Day). The last of these, at least, is still aptly named. It is a day to run around in rings, going to malls all over the galaxy. In your Saturn.

about Groundhog Day and Mother's Day and Secretary's Day—what if there just wasn't time any more?

So, I don't know. If it's all made up anyway, maybe we should all just come up with our own time and hang on to the things we know. Forget all that stuff about the favourite chair and the feelings of accomplishment and the obedient children. I'll take what I can get. A little light in the day, a little dark in the night, enough time to do my work and just get home before I fall asleep. Is that too much to ask?

I don't think so. I don't live far from work. Getting home only takes about forty-five minutes.

Replacement Parts

Oops.

My
mouse
is
busted.

I'm
stuck
on the
left
margin
.

Just
hold
on a
line or
two,
there's
a
compu

ter
shop
around
the
corner.

There. Sorry about that. It was a broken spring. The repairwoman said it was going to be too expensive to fix. She told me I'd be better buying a whole new mouse. I did. It cost me twenty-five bucks.

I find that worrisome. Not the money, but the idea. As an aging male with some fairly rusty springs myself, I think the matter deserves some discussion.

That little spring was a mechanical device. It's one of the few my computer has. I'm no mechanical whiz, myself. In fact, most of the time, when our Volkswagen blows a spring, I'd just as soon throw *it* out, too. But still, if it comes down to the mechanics versus the electronics, for me, there's no choice.

For one thing, mechanical things do not break down quietly. There are loud bangs, grinding gears and great columns of black, greasy smoke. It doesn't take a genius to know something is wrong, and, because of the grime and the sludge, not to mention the fingerprints, any mechanical transaction will leave a forensic trail that even a mechanical moron like me can eventually follow. Simply put, mechanics, and the things they fix, are lousy liars.

Electronics, on the other hand, are born to lie. They come in nondescript plastic boxes that pretend there is nothing going on inside of them. They break down without warning, or explanation, or guilt, and the people who come to fix them are quiet and antisocial and would rather be playing *Mortal Kombat*. They sit in your chair, at your desk, open your precious files and letters, break the springs in your mouse, tell you nothing about what went wrong in the first place, what they are doing to fix it or when it might happen again.

It's hard to believe we ever let them in the building. But while mechanics—both the people and the devices—have become a seriously endangered species, the demonic electronics have invaded, and conquered, every aspect of our lives.

At its most basic level, the true battleground for the mechanic/electronic conflict isn't the service station, or even the computer.

Think of playing golf. The eyes perceive the small, white ball below. The arms draw back the club, release, the legs and feet transfer weight in a subtle act of balance and *pow!* a beautiful, arcing drive sails forth, bounces once on the fairway and rolls onto the green. Pride fills the soul, the facial muscles relax and form a smile, and the legs happily carry the golfer forward further with a certainty of success. All mechanical systems are go.

Then, on the way to the next tee, the electronic department of the human being—that is, the conscious mind—boots up. "Hey!" it says with a flurry of brain impulses. "That's cool! Let me get in on that. Hold that club a little tighter! Watch your stance! Are you sure you know how to do this? There are people behind you, hurry up! Watch the ball! Watch the ball! Watch the ball! Oh, no, you moron! In the pond? What's the matter with you?"

Our mechanics don't stand a chance.

It wasn't always this way. When the majority of people survived or perished on the basis of their day-to-day physical stamina, our mechanics had to be taken seriously. But once we moved from the farm to the family room, and our mechanics embraced the idea of comfort and luxury over work and pain, the writing was on the wall. Now, with many of the major health problems of most North Americans stemming from inactivity, the mechanics have a hard time asserting their importance. Short of tipping back the La-Z-Boy and clicking the remote, there isn't a whole lot for them to do.

And while they sink deeper and deeper into their own cushy insignificance—second-guessing the stock markets, buying self-help manuals and trying to get a spot on "Oprah"—the electronics are having a field day. It's as if the geeks from the computer department snuck into head office and changed all the passwords.

I find myself thinking of Steve Austin.

He was the air force pilot played by Lee Majors in the 1970s hit TV series "The Six Million Dollar Man." Steve was flying an experimental craft, the show's opening sequence reminded us, when his ship suffered some sort of electro-mechanical failure and he was sent hurtling to the ground at the kind of speed that results in loud bangs and grinding gears and great columns of black, greasy smoke.

Steve didn't die, of course. There were still another forty-seven minutes of prime time drama and several years of reruns to go. But he was pretty banged up, with several key mechanical systems lost. This being the era preceding the twenty-five-dollar disposable mouse, however, the master surgeons of this imagined future decided Steve was worth rebuilding. They gave him replacement parts: an eye, an ear, and an arm and a leg that cost them just that, hence the name of the show.

Consequently, Steve Austin had amazing powers. He could run as fast as a speeding getaway van full of bad guys, throw those bad guys great distances and hear, beneath the soundtrack's cheesy, space-age sound effects, the sickening thud of their impact several counties away.

It was a pretty good idea for a TV show. After a few seasons, though, it became apparent that the producers had blown the budget rebuilding Steve and had nothing left in the pot to pay for decent writers or even acting lessons for the star.

But that wasn't the only problem with "The Six Million Dollar Man." In creating the show, it never occurred to anyone that the main character's mainframe might have benefited from a little refurbishing, too. Sure, Steve could throw hoods into the next area code, but imagine what his mind was saying while he was doing it. "Hold on a little tighter! Watch your stance! Hey! Listen to me! You're on TV!" What a lost opportunity. If they'd spent two or three million getting rid of that, they'd have had a *real* superhero, and they could have hired some real writers with the leftovers, too.

They didn't do that, of course. That is the kind of decision a mechanic would have made, and the electronics in charge, clearly, couldn't allow that. They might be bureaucratic and incompetent, but once they get hold of the reins of power, the electronics hang on as tightly as they do when they wreck a golf swing.

Think of business. The managers are in charge, and, since being in charge brings on a natural sense of entitlement, they keep hiring more management to make their jobs easier and themselves more important. This means the company is paying more and more salaries to people whose work doesn't earn the company any money. So, after a while, it's time to let somebody go. But who does management give the job of deciding whose jobs to cut? Why, other management, of course. They certainly couldn't trust anyone else to do it. Sometimes they even hire *more* management to help them out with the task. Naturally, those managers aren't going to point the finger at *their* managers. Doing that would only get them fired. Nor are they going to volunteer their own positions. So, after they have spent months (on astoundingly cushy salaries) studying the problem, they decide to fire the only people they can without firing themselves: the folks on the factory floor, the mechanics. This means the remaining few down there end up working harder, sometimes for even less money, and the company does even more poorly, while the electronics upstairs spend even more time playing *Mortal Kombat* and working on their terrible golf swings, until they are asked to take another look at what's going wrong.

So, here is my problem with all of this. I am thirty-seven years old. As I've noted many times, my own mechanics are long past their prime—about eleven years past, by most estimates—and are now working harder and harder, for less and less reward, than ever before, with no improvement in sight. On top of that, my electronics have realized that, by default, they now have the advantage and can start to really throw their weight around, wrecking golf swings and insisting on heart-pounding sprints at the end of otherwise pleasant workouts, until, eventually, defeated, one of the key mechanics—say, a hip—gives out completely.

"Don't worry!" the electronics cry. "We have solutions for that! Great minds have been working on it."

And they have. Doctors can now replace a person's hips, and they don't use bones or anything boring like that. Replacement hips are made of highly polished cobalt-chromium balls that connect to titanium alloy stems and are cemented into place with polymethylmethacrylate. Cool, eh? A person's electronics could stay busy working out how to say that for a good, long time, and that's just fine. It might shut them up while the mechanics learn to walk again.

That could work for the artificial knees, too, and the high-powered hearing aid, and the laser-surgery-assisted eyes. And, with any luck, by the time all that is installed, and great minds have improved things to the extent that those new, artificial limbs and senses are actually better than the old ones were, people will also be able to keep their blood (or hydraulic fluid, or whatever solution is needed by then) pumping happily, regardless of how much French pastry they have eaten, because they will have access to an artificial heart.

That window opened in 1982 with Robert Jarvik's artificial heart, the Jarvik-7. It was a miraculous thing, but there were problems in the end. The first person to receive one lived for only 112 days afterward. Subsequent patients did more poorly still, and didn't even survive long enough to watch very many episodes of "The Six Million Dollar Man."

But they are working on it. Great minds. They are rebuilding the body, one piece at a time, clearing the mechanics right off the factory floor. They are even prepared to replace themselves. Studies in artificial intelligence, the science charged with creating a replacement brain, are well under way, and while they face a daunting task, there is little question that they will eventually be up to it. And these new, brain-made brains will, I have no doubt, be even better at wrecking a golf swing (now performed with artificial arms, legs, hips, knees, etc.) than their creators were, and they will wonder, as their creators did, how they ended up with that nasty bug in the program that won't shut up while they're teeing off.

Not even that, however, will ever slow down the electronics in their inexorable quest for total control. Like those managers chosen to decide who gets fired, they have no alternative. It's a matter of survival. They are fighting the as yet still certain knowledge that no matter how great their achievements, and how many columns of black, greasy smoke their artificial bodies can create, in the end, their term in office must surely, and finally, end.

Upstairs, the office might be humming, with the data systems clicking over and new levels of Mortality being Kombatted with even more vigour. But when the last mechanic on the factory floor leaves his work station, goes to his locker, hangs up his hard hat, shuts down the lights and says goodbye, the breathing, the pumping, the living and the game, whether all players have defeated Goro or not, is over.

It seems a shame, to me, that it has to come to that. We're reasonable folks, mostly. All it would take is a little bit of patience and willingness to
compr
omise
and . . .

Damn.

Welcome To The Pleasure Dome

I didn't take much comfort from the recent interest in hairless men. Perhaps you missed it. I know it probably meant more to me than it did to, say, a man with long, thick, wavy hair. And by that I don't mean to discount it completely. It was nice to see women swooning over Patrick Stewart, and to know that all those hirsute brutes were shaving their heads and getting buzz-cuts to approximate the real thing. But for me it really would have been much better if it had happened about eighteen years ago, or anytime, for that matter, before that lovely spring day in Montreal when I went to get my hair cut.

I was nineteen. I was at the peak of my sexual appetite and abilities—at least, according to what I've read. If it was so, the only explanation I can fathom for the dizzying lack of activity in that department was a coinciding peak of naivete, social clumsiness and a tremendous knack for missing opportunity.

But it *was* a beautiful day. I had cash in my pocket and love on my mind, and inside I knew that a new haircut would be just the thing to have the women sunning themselves on the front steps of the university music building all aflutter as I sashayed by. So I went to the barbershop.

Well, no, I went to the hairstylist. There are differences. Namely, that there are no women in a barbershop except the ones in the girlie magazines found in the waiting area. My choice had more, I believe, to do with the aforementioned peak in naivete. There was something about the hairstylist's—the cursive lettering, the plants by the window, the lack of fat, smelly, former sailors spitting on fetid tiles caked with greasy old hair clippings—that suggested to me a greater likelihood that my new haircut would render the women all aflutter.

"How old are you?" the stylist asked. He was not particularly old, himself, and quite hairy, with long, thick, wavy hair that moved like a field of wheat in a summer breeze.

"Nineteen," I answered, as he inspected my head.

"Nineteen?" he roared incredulously. "You're bald!"

Of course, I *wasn't.*

I know, he was an expert in hair, someone who looked only at heads and hair and scalps all day long, and he had a much better view than I did of the crown of my head, where he suggested the outrageous thinning had already begun. I know all of that. I knew it then. But I wasn't prepared to think of myself as bald just yet. Especially when I later sashayed by the women on the steps of the music building and perceived no fluttering of any kind, or even any notice of my passing.

Like I said, if there had been a keen interest in hairless men at that time, or soon after, I would have taken much comfort from it. But there wasn't. At that time, the only bald men on the planet who were considered sexy in the least were Telly Savalas, who appealed to women my mother's age, and Burt Reynolds, who wore a toupee. Not much to make a young, apparently balding man optimistic.

At least, not in front of the music building. The science building, however, might have provided some encouragement. There were no women sunning themselves outside the science building, ever. But inside, I've since found out, there was plenty of the kind of information that would make a bald man stand at attention and take off his hat.

So if you, or someone you know, has just been deemed bald by a hairy hairstylist, and you are reeling with the accompanying dismay and self-doubt, or if you are a fully-furred man who has spent the past few paragraphs feeling entirely smug, please, read on.

BALDING FACT #1: The head of a balding man is just one big sex organ

In humans, hairless skin, such as is found on the lips and fingertips, has specialized nerve endings that are extremely sensitive. Hairy skin, however, requires the stimulation of the hair follicles. Now, I'll grant you, the top of my head is not as sensitive as my lips, nor quite as useful in an amorous situation, and it lacks the dexterity of my fingertips as well. Writing, for example, except for large, solid, oval figures made with a very large stamp pad, is right out. But by the time the still-crowned heads of my generation are just beginning to approach the baldness challenge, my dome will have been hairless for long enough that it will, I remain confident, be able to write a love sonnet, recite it and collect the appropriate reward.

BALDING FACT #2: Men go bald because they are destined to enjoy delicious sex scandals and never get caught

One of the major purposes of hair in the natural world is camouflage. Evolution has very efficiently encouraged those animals whose pattern of hair has given them, and their offspring, some advantage in the survival and procreation game. One only has to think of the tiger's stripes helping it to remain hidden in the tall grasses of its hunting ground, or of the shiny, greenish coat of the three-toed sloth concealing it in the dense foliage of the tropical rain forest. But the jungles of the human world are not green, leafy or grassy. They are the boardrooms of political power and the trading floors of the financial district. Take a look one day along Bay Street or Wall Street, or at the crowd leaving the Houses of Parliament at two in the afternoon after a busy working day. A forest of tall, thick, bouffant coiffures with cowlicks and ducktails? I should say not. Such fools only draw attention to themselves.

Quickly, now, think of two very rich and powerful bald men who have been publicly ridiculed for their foolish sexual dalliances and written about extensively in such esteemed publications as *People* magazine. Right. There aren't any. While furry fools like Gary Hart and Bill Clinton keep getting caught with their hairless areas of highly sensitive skin going where it will only get them in trouble, the balding elite blend into the crowd and enjoy their pleasures, whatever they may be, far from any glare at all, save from their own scalps.

BALDING FACT #3: Balding men have more active brains

Throughout nature, the main role of hair in the life of a mammal is protection against heat loss. The exposed scalp, therefore, with its natural cooling system of cutaneous circulation, is clearly nature's way of countering the risk of overheating in the balding male's feverishly active mind. This is the equivalent of a very powerful computer requiring a high-speed fan to keep it functioning at optimal levels.

Obviously, a man with a great deal of hair on his head must not have a whole lot going on upstairs.

On the other hand, a thin fringe of hair around the sides and back of the head is generally referred to as a Hippocratic Wreath. Which great thinker, teacher and philosopher gave *his* name to a hairstyle employing a full head of hair? *Have* there been any great thinkers with a full head of hair?

Okay, Einstein. But in most portraits it looks as though he's either trying to pull it out or let it die from lack of care.

BALDING FACT #4: Women don't care about the hair on a man's head

Well, all right, perhaps they do. But subconsciously, there is another level of interest and appreciation going on that would make a barber blush. It has nothing to do with gleaming scalps or long, flowing locks. It has to do with smell.

In the course of my work on the CBC Radio program "Fresh Air," I had the tremendous pleasure of meeting George Bubenik, an endocrinologist and a professor of physiology at the University of Guelph. Professor Bubenik told me that for all mammals, including humans, the business of mate selection is largely determined by pheromones.

Pheromones are airborne chemicals released by a number of animal and plant species, and a few insects, to communicate specific information to other members of the species. These messages, whether consciously or not, are perceived through smell. Dogs, for example, distribute pheromones when they pee, to let other dogs know they have claimed a given hydrant or tree as their own. There are also alarm pheromones, which many species use to warn their fellow dogs, fish, grasshoppers or fire hydrants that there is a predator, or a dog, present.

Trees even use alarm pheromones. Dr. Bubenik told me that many different kinds of trees send out alarm pheromones when they have been attacked by parasites. They are warning their neighbours. Being trees, however, I'm not sure quite what those neighbours do, exactly, with the information. Certainly, in evolutionary terms, running away must still be a long way off.

But it is not the job of the pheromones to question the value or usefulness of their message. Like the Home Shopping Network, they just keep broadcasting, whether anyone's buying or not. And believe me, they don't just have their eye on that nice fella or gal by the water cooler. He or she would be fine, to be sure—but who's that across the street? Look over there in the coffee shop! On the subway! Pheromones are not choosy; they have a product to sell and they are selling hard. Come on baby! Whooee! Priced to move!

Despite the valiant efforts of our many deodorants, detergents, soaps, body gels, apricot scrubs, toilet waters and colognes, humans are constantly sending out pheromones. In one sense, they are performing a very important procreational function. Pheromones tell potential mates whether they are genetically well matched, and if their pairing would be likely to produce healthy and balanced children. But that doesn't make them respectable in any civilized sense. They are maniacs. They don't care where they are or who it is they've just met, or even whether there isn't an affordable hotel in the neighbourhood. They want sex and they want it now. Anywhere, any place, any time.

The only exception to this rule is among pregnant women. Women still send out pheromones when pregnant, but they are no longer the hard-sell, hubba-hubba variety. Those pheromones have won the company sales prize and have been sent on leave to the Caribbean for at least nine months. In their place, the home-front pheromones call off the smelly males and start broadcasting a niche-market program for people that smell like extended family. They are looking for some help to raise the kids. This system is based on the still embarrassingly all-too-accurate assumption that once insemination has occurred, the male of the species will take the first available subway all the way across town.

Pheromones are secreted from scent glands located among the hair follicles at the intersection of the limbs and the trunk—the crotch and the armpits. The more hair, the more smell. The more smell, the stronger the sales pitch, and—naivete, social clumsiness and missed opportunity aside—the greater the chance of winning the company prize.

Now (says the balding author, warming to his point), I honestly haven't done any scientific study on this, but it doesn't take much more than a glance around the average health club change room to tell you that most bald men have more than their share of fur on areas other than their heads. If you are a man, you'll know this to be true and will join me in reaching the obvious conclusion about those of us lucky enough to be bald. If you're a woman, you could poke your head in the dressing room and look for yourself, or just go nosing around the next time you pass the water cooler.

> BALDING FACT #5: Male pattern baldness is caused by hormonal imbalances, specifically, excessive levels of testosterone

Ho hum, eh? The stuff that makes a man a man is also what makes him go bald. So what? I've already proven scientifically that bald men are more likely to be involved in wonderful and undetected sex scandals, that we are smarter, more attractive and genetically selected to procreate at a more feverish pace, and that we can write poems not just in our heads, but *with* our heads. Who cares about a little testosterone? Do we really need to be any more attractive?

But I didn't know any of that eighteen years ago on that lovely spring day. I was not studying science or, in any formal sense, procreation. I was studying music, the industry that, at the time, was giving us the bountiful hairlines of Gino Vannelli, Rod Stewart (who isn't related to Patrick) and Gene Simmons, of the band Kiss, who even then was reputed to have bedded thousands of women, taken each one's photograph and kept all of those snapshots in an enormous album—sort of a hairy bachelor's brag book.

By that time, hairiness had been a hit for close to fifteen years, and, despite the mess on everyone's shoulders, no one saw any thinning in sight. Surgeons who performed hair transplants, with endorsements from hockey stars, were harvesting fees like rows of corn and leaving their patients with the stubble. In the mid-1980s, pharmaceutical firms trumpeted the discovery of Minoxidil, a drug originally designed for hypertension that was found to slow hair loss in many cases, and in a few, actually to grow new hair on already balding areas. The only way to test it, though, is to try it. If you do, you have to smear the stuff on your head every day. A year's worth costs close to $1,000, and, if you decide to spend the rest of your savings on a whirlwind tour to show off your new locks, you'd better not forget the Minoxidil at home. Soon after the daily ablutions fall off, so does the hair.

But back then, who cared? It was hair for the pulling, and in the fight against balding, nothing was against the rules.

Even the offices of power got brushed into the fray: 1980 saw Pierre Trudeau and René Lévesque, both brilliant statesmen (and no slouches in the procreative area, either) battling each other on the issues of federalism, bilingualism, education, domestic policy and the very future of Canada and Quebec. Yet, curiously, they agreed on hairstyle. Both were bald, and, fooling no one, opted for the old grow-it-long-on-one-side-and-flop-it-over-the-top ruse. They were covered by the press from sea to sea, the glare of attention bringing even greater shine to the gaps in the heartland of each man's cranial constituency.

Then the crash came. Marlon Brando appeared shaved clean in *Apocalypse Now*. Popular music's new rave was a balding math teacher look-alike named Phil Collins. Cybill Shepherd fell for Bruce Willis, Kelsey Grammer got his own TV show, and the Duchess of York was photographed topless with a balding man, not her husband, sucking on her toes.

And, at the front of this shining pack, steering at warp nine through the asteroid belts of mop-headed producers and intergalactic bad guys alike, with nary a drop of perspiration (let alone Minoxidil) on his almost hairless head, was, as Captain Jean-Luc Picard of the starship *Enterprise*, the actor at the apex of all alopecia, Patrick Stewart.

Previous versions of the "Star Trek" series had done well with male audiences, but "The Next Generation" became a huge money-maker primarily by engaging an entirely new audience quadrant: women. Some analysis said women liked the show's emphasis on relationships over violence; others cited the fact that, for the first time, female characters had a greater role in the action—both valid points. But most of the success of the show eventually came to rest squarely on the uncluttered head of Picard. He was brave, he was reasonable, he avoided violence without being cowardly, he was caring without being cloying, and, amazingly, he was bald.

Speaking as an asteroid trailing near the tail end of the demographic comet that is the postwar baby boom, I do wonder about that a little bit. With all due respect to Mr. Stewart and his acting aplomb, the whole thing does seem like slightly more than a coincidence. By 1990, most of the boomers who were going to go bald already had. In retrospect, it doesn't seem like much of a surprise to find that thick, wavy hair was deemed less interesting at the precise time when close to half the men in the population didn't have any any more.

And, science and pheromones aside, I would have to question how well the trickle-down effect works in this case. I have yet to meet a bald man, for example, who, once "Star Trek: The Next Generation" had reached its peak in popularity, found himself pushing away beautiful women.

Despite all of that, and my dismal non-fluttering failure that spring day on the steps of the music building, and the accuracy of that hairstylist's assessment of my follicles' future, I did eventually manage to overcome enough of my enduring knack for naivete, social clumsiness and missed opportunity to cobble together a passable youth. And as to whether my balding aided or abetted, who can say?

Besides, there's another reason I'm not sure I want to know.

Male pattern baldness is handed down genetically. The chrome-dome chromosome[1] can be passed on by either the mother or the father, but it's the young man's hormones, released at puberty, that combine with his genes to determine ultimately how much shine there is up top.

---

[1] It's a gene, actually. I just liked the rhyme.

So, even if that genetic information is only part of the equation, it still has to take some of the responsibility for turning what used to be a fine, fully-haired and polite young man into the hot-blooded, pheromone-spewing, skirt-chasing wag that we've already established he is once he begins to lose his hair.

So, what does that say about his parents? Or his grandparents?

When he was my age, my father's hairline was exactly like mine. I knew my mom's dad a little, and never met my father's, and now they're both dead, but I've seen pictures. There isn't a lot of hair on either one, and there wasn't for much of their adult lives, either.

So, I don't know. I don't think I'd be too comfortable talking to my mom about how much of my raging sex drive I can blame on her, or her father. I'm just now getting to know my dad well enough to maybe make a joke about it sometime in the next decade. And if my grandfathers were still alive, it mightn't be the easiest thing to bring up with them, either.

What we'd need, I think, to really find out, is somewhere to meet and talk. Just a place with a few chairs, maybe some magazines, and the radio on. The kind of place a bunch of guys could go on a Saturday morning and warm up to difficult questions over a few days, or weeks, without feeling any pressure. If there were a barber chair in the place, I guess that wouldn't hurt. It would give us something to do, even if none of us had any hair. Somehow, at thirty-seven, I don't think a couple of fat sailors, or the fetid, greasy tiles, would bother me that much any more.

Besides, it's a funny thing about barber chairs. With

those arms, and the headrest, and the way they swivel around so easily, once you're sitting in one, with your trusted mates all around, it's easy to imagine you're not a customer in a barbershop at all but the captain on the bridge of a starship. With a crew like that, and so much brain activity and history on our side, we could conquer the universe. But I think I'd start with a visit to that nice little planet out in the Alderon Quadrant, first. The one where the inhabitants are hairless and ageless and rarely have trouble talking to their ancestors about difficult questions because they're so smart and perceptive. And, best of all, they communicate by smell.

Leisure & Pleasure, Leisure & Seizure

Webster's Dictionary says leisure is "time free from work or duties."

I can remember what felt like endless hours in my teenage years in which I did absolutely nothing but wish that time would pass. It's not that I didn't have work to do. Grade ten chemistry comes to mind as something that might have benefited from a little more time away from the leisure lab. But for a teenager, school and chores and anything else that the adult world might consider meaningful work are, in fact, leisure activities. The adolescent's full-time job is growing up. The assignments, the criteria for success and the evaluation process can all change at a moment's notice, and, regardless of performance or knowledge or ambition, there is one obstacle to the job's completion that simply cannot be avoided: the necessary passage of time.

Contrary to the romantic visions of youth often conjured by romantic former youths, the only time an adolescent ever seizes the day is to throw it out and get on to the next one.

And then the job of adolescence is done, and a new assignment takes over: finding time.

If time is money, then young adulthood and middle age are spent in abject poverty, squandering time to make money, which is actually time, so it is time spent to make time, which costs still more time, which leaves nothing.

It's amazing to me that we even find the time to get older—perhaps, instead, time finds us. When it does, age sets in, and the time market is flooded. The currency is suddenly devalued, and the brokers and tellers and bank managers have all gone home for a glass of warm milk and a mid-afternoon nap.

It is hard for me to imagine how it will feel to suddenly have more time than I know what to do with. When I think of my senior years now, I see golden days full of ambition. I see practising my trombone enough to be as good as I should have been long ago. I see working on the jump shot I wish I had but have never had the time to learn. I see spending the time with my children that, these days, I too often let slip away. On really bad days, I even see redoing grade ten chemistry.

But the truth is, right now, in the time bear market known as middle age, when I do, by some small miracle, end up with an hour or two, I don't do any of those things, even though there is often no reason I couldn't. I am too dumbstruck by the luxury of nothing to do. I go to the hardware store and look at nothing. I stand at the window in the back room and try to remember moments I said I would never forget. I sit on the front porch and drink coffee and try to imagine the days when that will be all I have to do.

In fact, when I really think about it, I can't imagine why that habit would be likely to change much in twenty-five years' time. And that brings forward an uncomfortable conclusion: that youth is spent daydreaming about adulthood, adulthood spent daydreaming about the senior years, and the senior years spent daydreaming about the previous two.

Because time abhors a vacuum, and I don't particularly want to see all my future leisure time seized and sucked into the dustbuster of everyday life, I have set one goal I know I will truly enjoy meeting. It will work only if my children, once they reach middle age, turn out anything at all like me. But I have already seen them daydreaming an awful lot, and I don't think that's too much of a stretch. I promise, when I finally have some time, I'll get together with my children, perhaps to make music or play basketball, but mostly to spend a whole lot of time sitting on the front porch, or staring out the window in the back room, or wandering together around the hardware store, remembering all the fun things we did when none of us had any time.

Round Dance

One night in March 1997, I heard a sound that sent me back to my student days.

I went to school in Boston for two years, in the early 1980s. They were good years for a few of that city's venerable institutions. One was Boston College, a Jesuit school with a campus of squat, Gothic buildings, nestled into the western suburbs. Their basketball team was rather squat in those days, too. The marquee player was a six-foot guard named John Bagley. In any other profession (except furnace repair), to be six feet tall would usually be considered an asset. But in American college basketball, being only six feet tall is the equivalent of being a three-storey walk-up tendering a bid for a new helipad across the street from the Pan Am Building. John Bagley and Boston College made it to the fourth round of the championship in 1982. Bagley averaged twenty-two points per game, and for several mad days that spring, he carried the city on his shoulders.

Also that spring, the now tired but then glorious Boston Celtics of the NBA shook the dust out of their mean and nasty (and a little bit squat) old home, Boston

Garden, with a riveting season of their own. With the likes of Larry Bird and Robert Parrish, that gritty edition of the Celtics had one championship tucked into their shorts from the year before and missed a second chance only by the merest inches in a cruel and harrowing seven-game conference final with the Philadelphia 76ers.

But I didn't know anything about basketball when I moved to Boston. I was there to study music. My main interest was another of Boston's venerable institutions: the Boston Symphony Orchestra and their elegant home, Symphony Hall.

Symphony Hall is one of the best places in the world to hear music. You can feel the building's warmth from the moment you step inside. Whether there is one musician on stage or one hundred, you can hear every note from every seat, and, as many musicians have been known to admit in private, Symphony Hall has the magic gift of honouring the most beautiful sounds, no matter how tiny, while somehow simultaneously obscuring the bad ones, no matter how huge.

The place was built in 1900. It has lived through countless shifts in artistic temperament (from Leroy Anderson to Béla Bartók) and is as full of history as Boston is full of beans. There is a plaque in the foyer that commemorates the musicians on board the *Titanic* for putting music above survival as they continued to play while the ship modulated steadily downward. The main section of raked seating on the orchestra level is removable. It takes about twenty-five workers and they can do the job overnight, replacing the seats with café tables for the Boston Pops Concerts, turning one of the world's most cherished rooms for the enjoyment of serious music into a giant nightclub. And, all around the upper level, the main hall boasts porticos that house statues of Greek deities, all naked and anatomically correct. At several points in the city's puritanical past, various prominent prudes complained about them. There was even talk of removing them, until it was pointed out that they, and their housing (if not their attire), were part of the Great Hall's acoustic design, and that any alteration would have a detrimental effect on the sound. Modesty and civility were fine and good, Boston's upper crust decided, but if they got in the way of good music, then to hell with them.

I worked as an usher at Symphony Hall to make extra money while I went to school. The pay wasn't great, but, as part of my compensation, I heard so many recitals I can't remember them all. There was Isaac Stern, Andres Segovia, Ella Fitzgerald and Tommy Flanagan, Rudolf and Peter Serkin, Joan Baez and a whole season of the wonderful Boston Symphony Orchestra.

The other perk of the job was that I could go backstage. This gave me access to a great number of opportunities, such as being ignored by jazz singer Joe Williams when I told him how much I'd enjoyed his concert. He'd just finished slathering two thousand people with oozing charm, even asking them to sing the *ooh-ooh* part in a Billy Joel song, but he didn't even look at me. He just bit into another chicken finger. There were, however, great experiences, too. There was a peephole on the rear wall of the stage. From there I saw Kurt Masur dance mesmerizing performances of Brahms out of the orchestra, and watched the late Klaus Tennstedt, in an unforgettable Beethoven's Fifth, cue the French horns as though he were whipping a team of mules.

But the greatest part about going backstage at Symphony Hall was the downstairs musician's lounge, which we called the lunchroom. The lunchroom was the one place where Boston Garden, Boston College and Symphony Hall found their common ground. Bostonians, I discovered, especially musical ones, are mad for basketball.

The scene in the lunchroom during basketball season was nothing short of surreal. The musicians practically ran down there during concert intermissions. Studious, white-haired string players in white ties and tails, who had only minutes before been coaxing a tone as soft as butter from a Mozart serenade, sat glued to the television, whooping like wild men or throwing down their mangled vending machine coffee cups in disgust. As the season went on, the personnel manager had to page them five or six times over the intercom to get them back on stage for the second half. Once, during the playoffs, to groans of disappointment, he actually had to come downstairs and turn the TV off himself.

On the surface, it was hard to see the connection between music and basketball. I'm sure none of those musicians had ever played ball. Most wouldn't even work in the yard for fear of injuring their hands. But one day, in a music history class, our professor told us about an idea Johann Kepler had, back in the late 1500s.

Johann Kepler was a mathematician who was the first to accurately describe how human beings see, and what happens to light after it has entered a telescope. In a mere seven years he went from being a theology student who'd never finished his studies to Imperial Mathematician of the Holy Roman Empire, in 1594. Kepler was also an astronomer who wrote extensively on the movement of the planets. His Three Principles of Planetary Motion hold to this day.

I'd be lying if I told you I understood any of them. Kepler's Principles weren't on the exam in my music history course. What we cared about was a much earlier theory of his.

This idea began with another great astronomer, Nicolaus Copernicus, who had died in 1543. Copernicus believed that the (then) six planets[1] could be grouped into giant, hollow, invisible globes that regulated their orbits. Copernicus called these globes Spheres.

Kepler's big interest, some fifty years later, was finding an order and harmony to the movement of the planets. If there were Spheres rotating in the heavens, Kepler reasoned, in the same way a finger produces music when it traces the rim of a wine glass, the movements of those Spheres, and the resulting vibrations, would produce sound. If those sounds were ordered, it would create a kind of harmony, a series of celestial chords, which he called the Music of the Spheres.

This theory is usually introduced into music history classes as a warning that the best days of the music profession, in terms of its value to the general population, have passed. Under the theory of the Music of the Spheres, if a person fell ill, they were thought to be out of tune with the universe. Therefore, to be cured, they needed the services not of a fancy, self-important downtown doctor who sees hundreds of patients every day and drives a Mercedes, but of a musician. In fact, for a while, musicians

---

[1] He would likely have favoured the thirty-day month made up of five, six-day weeks, I'm guessing.

were actually referred to as physicians, because of their healing powers. We don't know, however, whether in those days the organization now referred to as the OMA (Ontario Medical Association) would have actually been the Ontario Musicians' Association, or whether it would have had enough clout to threaten the government with the horrific prospect of a shortage of emergency cellists in Timmins. Somehow I doubt it. In fact, the only true links remaining between the two types of physicians are an obsession with money (either in lack or in surplus) and, in some cases, an interest in pharmaceuticals.

Nevertheless, Kepler's Music of the Spheres is still taught in select music history classes, even if only with a "those were the days" sensibility. If the teacher is a very complete and entertaining one, as mine was, he or she will elaborate on this topic only to inform the students that the theory of Heavenly Spheres is utter rot. The universe, my teacher told us, is not divided into spheres; it is an unimaginable empty space cluttered with chunks of rock of various sizes that fly around according to their own and each other's gravitational forces, with almost no larger order at all. If you're hearing music on a clear, starry night, he told us, it is because you are passing a nightclub.

But during those concert intermissions down in the lunchroom at Symphony Hall, I had to wonder about that. Those white-haired string players had incredible ears. And when they watched basketball, they didn't go wild for the slam-dunks and alley-oops. It was the ball they loved to watch, that fat, orange sphere, as big as Jupiter, shot from thirty feet out and floating through the air to the basket, or soaring over the key in the hands of Julius Irving, until he placed it in the hoop as gently as if it were an egg.

There is something ethereal about the way a ball moves. Locomotion for humans is so awkward. Even if you are Julius Irving, you still have to step from one foot to another on those gangly twigs we call legs. But a sphere in motion shows no effort at all. It is a thing born to move, over land or through the air. For a sphere, crossing the simplest distance is an act of beauty, and that motion is everywhere in our world. Kids with a baseball or hipsters in the pool hall. Tennis courts and racquet sports and pinball in shopping malls.

To me, the most reverent spherical exchange of all is a simple game of catch. Have you ever noticed how little people talk when they are playing catch? It's actually a very awkward thing to do. The talk is broken and disjointed and only gets in the way, because it's unnecessary. People who are playing catch don't need to talk. They're already communicating.

And if spherical objects flying through the air can be said to have an ethereal, even spiritual significance, then sixteen years after my history lesson on Kepler, on a cold, clear night in March, I can claim to have attended services in the Temple of Spherical Worship.

My neighbour, Ron, was my guide. Ron is a golfer. By the time winter finally dribbles to a stop, and little shoots of green begin to poke up through the garden, and the crisp mornings of fall seem about as far back as Copernicus, Ron gets itchy. So, does Ron book a trip to Florida? Heck, no. Ron goes to the Golf Dome.

The Golf Dome is just north of Toronto. It is an inflatable building made of bright, white plastic. It is about a hundred yards wide, a soccer-field-sized soccer ball, buried up to its waist. You may cringe, and I wouldn't blame you, at the idea of putting a building that is essentially a big, air-filled bag in the same piece of writing that earlier attempted to capture the beauty of Symphony Hall, or even Boston Garden, but bear with me. Inside the Golf Dome there is a pro shop, and a waiting room with a big-screen TV that plays only the Golf Channel. There is a putting green and a few, small sand traps. And, through a rotating door, there are forty-six little confessional-like cubicles where people stand in front of a small patch of astroturf, with a golf club in hand and a bucket full of golf balls at their sides. The folks at the Golf Dome stay in those booths for hours at a time, whaling golf balls out into the big empty room. The turf below ends up looking like the living-room rug after an encounter with a box full of packing chips.

People will tell you that they play golf for the exercise, or for the pleasure of walking on grass and the feeling of being outdoors on a nice day. But I say balls to that. It's the Music of the Spheres. The Golf Dome faithful aren't always swinging. They stop and watch for minutes at a time, looking up and out, and listening to the rain of little white planets arcing out over the carpet and off into artificial space.

The Golf Dome has fifty thousand golf balls in supply. It is the full-time job of two employees just to collect them all and bring them back. The night I was there it was a kid of maybe eighteen who had the pleasure. He drove a small tractor that looked like a rider-mower, with a kind of rolling lobster trap to catch the balls and a protective cage around the cockpit. That's an occupational precaution, I guess. I mean, if you take forty-six winter-weary golfers, fifty thousand balls and nothing to aim at, even if the place is a shrine, well, most golfers aren't saints. Even I tried to hit him.

It was kind of a low point for me. For all the sanctity of the place, and all the worship that goes on inside, I remained unmoved. I guess maybe the Music of the Spheres in the Golf Dome wasn't ethereal enough for me.

I am getting somewhere on the basketball court, though. I started playing a while ago. It was years after I'd moved away from Boston, and, strangely enough, after I'd given up playing music professionally, too. But somehow the euphoria of those spherically crazed string players stayed with me. I play once a week, now, in a church gym that is so small you can't throw a three-pointer without hitting the fire alarm on the ceiling. But it is a lot of fun. It's a chance to run around with a bunch of aging hackers like me. Now and then I sink a shot and afterwards we all go out and put back all the pounds we just ran off by drinking beer and watching basketball on TV.

It was after one of those games, in March 1997, with my basketball buddies, and, coincidentally, just after my trip to the Golf Dome, that I heard that lovely sound I'd long forgotten. It was March Madness time—the American college basketball championships. The final game between Arizona and Kentucky was a classic, tense to the end, with most of the winning points scored on foul shots —long, slow, arcing throws from the top of the key, with moments of silence as the ball travelled through space.

It was close to midnight when Arizona finally won, and a cold, clear night as I walked home. I looked up into the night sky, and for a moment I thought I was back in the Golf Dome. The stars were out; even through Toronto's smog, there were easily fifty thousand. And low in the sky in the northwest, like a 3-wood drive still on the rise, was one of those chunks of rock that fly around the universe. It was Hale-Bopp, the comet that visited that winter, shared a little of our gravity and, well, lessened a little of it, too. There it was, arcing silently across the sky, without a net or an artificial carpet or even a kid on a tractor in sight.

I stood still and watched for I don't know how long. The traffic was noisy, but, you know, I listened, and I'd swear I heard music.

Look Out Below

My parents live in what used to be the family cottage. It's north of Montreal on a small lake, which is really just a detour in a lazy river, and the water tends to be a little murky. One summer a few years ago, though, for some reason, it was unusually clear.

I have spent hundreds of hours with that water—swimming in it, standing up to my neck in it during the heat wave in '75, and, mostly, canoeing on it, in a fifteen-foot canvas/cedar canoe I bought with my paper route money when I was in high school. I love that canoe. It's light and fast and absolutely perfect for one person on a murky lake who finds himself with nothing to do. I often consider bringing it back to Toronto after we've been visiting. Lord knows Lake Ontario is murky, too. I tell myself that if the canoe were right there in the garage I might be moved to take it down for a paddle now and then.

But I always leave it behind. It's an eight-hour drive from my parents' place. Once push comes to drive and the trunk is stuffed, the kids are loaded in and we're ready to go, I never have the heart. That canoe lives there. It wouldn't be right to take it anywhere else.

So, I cherish the few moments I have with that water

and that canoe on our summer visits. I have a standard route: around the point, through the narrows, under the bridge, portage over the road or, if the water is low enough but not too low, through the giant culvert and back around the long fifth basin and home.

That summer when the water was so clear, the first free moment I had I was out in the canoe, but I didn't get very far. It was strange for me to be looking down and actually seeing something other than slate grey, or dancing sunlight, or myself. There were reeds down there, and all kinds of gullies and hollows on the bottom. I'd never seen any of it before. It made me wonder if Narcissus might have ended up a marine biologist if he'd just had a clearer pond.

I finally made it to the point before the narrows, a mere thirty yards from our dock, when, determined to press on, I looked down one last time, and I saw them: fish. At first, there were just a few little guys—perch and sunfish. But then I saw a bass, and a fat little doré. In Ontario they call them pickerel, but I like the Quebec name, doré. It means golden, because of the colour of their bellies. And it's true, I could see the flash of gold as it turned. But I guess that's a blessing as well as a curse. Once the sun hit that doré it got out of there fast, and, sure enough, right behind was a huge, dark shape that looked like a pike. It slid through the shadow of the canoe so quickly I couldn't be sure, but whatever it was, it was after the doré, and it was big. All I really saw was a pair of eyes and a snout, but those jaws were open, and I could almost count the teeth.

That was as far as I canoed that day. I stayed in that spot, watching, for the rest of the morning.

It was vindication of a kind for me. The old Hungarian

couple from across the narrows spend a lot of time around that spot, just off the point and before the narrows. The place has a reputation for fish. No one says that, of course, but I see them out there, early in the morning, chugging pensively by in their runabout, lips pursed, cardigans buttoned, trolling lines and watching.

I'd spent my time fishing there, too, as a teenager—hours and hours and hours. I preferred casting from the shore, at dusk. I'd bring an old paint can with a smoke fire in it to keep the blackflies off, step in as far as I could with my big wellingtons and cast forever, just watching that lure fly out and come back over and over again. It's a delightful feeling, the easy repetition of casting followed by the satisfying plunk of the lure on the lake. I enjoyed it no matter what I caught, which was good, because I caught only one fish. One. A medium-sized pike. Every evening of every summer of my entire youth, with a fishing rod in my hand, and that was it: one fish.

Except during the heat wave of '75.

I'm always astounded by the temperatures in that place. In the winter it can be so cold the propane turns to liquid one day and hot enough to turn off the furnace the next. The summers are usually bland by comparison, but the summer of '75 wasn't.

It was the last summer before Canada went to the metric system. Maybe the sun decided to see if it could hit triple digits one last time, I don't know, but the mercury in our old Fahrenheit thermometer stayed above ninety for over a week, and by noon, most days, it was well over one hundred. The air was like cotton and the lake was like soup. Even the flies didn't bother biting after a while.

One evening I decided the physical exertion of casting

a lure for a few minutes might be enough to get me to sleep that night, despite the thirty-pound funk that was suspended in the air over my bed, and I trudged down to the point.

My first cast went about ten feet and snagged a log. Ten minutes later, my second went twelve feet and snagged another. My third finally had some distance, but when I snagged again, I almost left the rod there and walked away.

Then the snag moved. At least, I thought it might have. It wasn't really a pull. It felt more like something tipping over under the water. I began to reel it in, still not sure what it was but feeling more and more that it must be a log, or a tire, because I felt like I was dragging it along the mud on the bottom.

As I dragged it into the shallows, it felt even heavier. The lake was thick and still. There hadn't been enough wind to dry a hanky in a week. When the end of the line was no more than ten feet out, in about a foot of water, I saw the merest ripple on the surface. That was the warning. The tug that followed almost snapped the rod.

The water boiled. Something broke the surface. It might have been part of a pike's tail, but it looked more like a shovel. Either way, I couldn't really look because I was losing the rod. My hands had been sweaty for a week and would have been lucky to get a grip on sandpaper, let alone some lake monster that wanted to take me water-skiing. I had about an inch more clearance on my wellingtons before they turned into wading pools. I gave one mighty pull with all the strength I could find and suddenly found myself on my keester in the soupy lake, with the fishing line tangled in the bushes beside me.

It had chewed through the line and kept my favourite lure—a silver Smorgasbord. I saw it flash as the thing swam away.

I told the old Hungarian man about it the next time he chugged by. "The pike," he said, with a tiny smile. I couldn't tell if he was laughing at me or not.

After that, I never had another nibble. For all I knew, in the years that followed, even the tadpoles had left that lake.

Until I saw all those fish that summer the water was clear. I spent every spare minute of that vacation watching the fish. I even ditched my cherished canoe. It was too much work to keep it still once the wind came up. I tried the pedal boat, too, but the paddle scared them off. The best vehicle for fish-watching, I found, was an air mattress. The wide, flat surface made a shady pool they liked to gather in. I could lie in the sun and enjoy the show: bright colours, flashes of gold, graceful, balletic movements. It was public entertainment of the finest kind.

Within my family, however, my own public image was taking a bit of a thrashing. Young children are a lot of work at a country place like that. Ours were three and one at the time, each with a nose for trouble and the attention span of a rock bass. With the canoe, I could at least entertain one of them for a while, but spending hours drifting silently by myself thirty yards from the dock, after a day or two, was becoming understandably difficult to justify. I mean, to them, it looked as though I was just lying around.

And then, in the clear waters off the point, I saw something that would prove I had a reason to be out there all along. Something even more entrancing than all those fish. Down there between the reeds, among the hollows and gullies and minnows and guppies, I'll swear it's true, I began to see dollar signs.

Think about it. The leisure industry is in turmoil. Movies and travel have been up and down. Tourism is either dying or flying, depending on the dollar. The boomers are aging and they're looking for something moderately athletic that won't remind them of all the other much more athletic things they used to do that they can't really do any more. The one sporting activity that has enjoyed consistent growth in the past few years is bird-watching, and it isn't hard to figure out why. It appeals to the ecological conscience without hurting industry. It involves fitness, but no one's going to need to be carried out on a stretcher. It's perfect.

So, why not fish-watching?

They've tried it before. Remember the high-rolling 1980s? Real estate tycoons were flipping condos like flapjacks and junk bond dealers were dropping entire countries when the yen had a bad day. Talk about stress! When those people came home and kicked off their tassel-loafers, they needed to relax. So, they installed aquariums the size of BMWs in their studies and spent the evenings throwing mice to the piranhas.

And, of course, there's whale-watching.

I went whale-watching once. It was a cold and windy October day on the Bay of Fundy, and the water was so choppy the inside of your mouth would turn green just watching the dock. We spent an hour and a half out on the heaving brine, steaming after distant spouts with our hands in our pockets and our stomachs in our armpits. Most of us were thinking we would have been better off spending our money on a roll of Tums and rental copies of the complete films of David Cronenberg.

Then we saw one. A fin whale surfaced right behind our boat. It was the size of a small train. We'd all been flying here and there, lunging for cameras and spyglasses and barf bags, but when that whale slipped by, we all fell silent. Its eye was as big as a softball and I'd swear it was looking right at me. My bones lined up. I felt as if I'd spoken with someone from another planet. I'll never forget it.

From a marketing point of view, though, whale-watching has problems. If you're going to really rake in the barnacles, you've got to reach the mainstream. Vomit and hypothermia might be big with the tree-huggers, but they don't play in the suburbs. And to turn any more than a fin on a fin whale, you have to get the volume up. I've seen those giant whale-watching excursions in the tourist centres along the coast. There are billboards for miles. The boats look like space shuttles. If the intimacy of whale-watching is the selling point, most of those people, and their whales, are completely missing the boat.

The biggest problem, from a purely business point of view, however, is the level of emotion involved. All that intense communication with an intelligent species gets pretty demanding for the average Joe. But with fish-watching, there's none of that. There are smart fish, I'm sure, but I think for most of us a relationship with a fish would have to be considered "marrying down."

Fish-watching: it's easy, it's free, and there's a market just waiting for it. If nothing else, you could clean up on all those fair-weather birders who have jumped on the bandwagon. Really, how many of them actually look forward to freezing early mornings and burrs in their socks?

Fish-watching gives them the same thrilling encounter with nature while they float around in the midday sun, lounging on an air mattress!

Guidebooks, paraphernalia, sponsorships . . . out there off the point at my parents' place, the more I thought about it, the more I was convinced. With fish-watching, all I had to do was open the net and the dollars would come swimming right in.

There was only one hitch. I don't think too many birders have to suppress the urge to grab that evening grosbeak, roll it in flour and fry it up for lunch. That's right. I'm ashamed to admit it, after all the pleasure they gave me, but gazing down at those fish for all that time, I started wanting to eat them. There was no good reason for it. We weren't short of food, and I sure wasn't looking forward to cleaning them. But still, the urge wouldn't go away.

A day or so later I was driving back from town with my three-year-old son, and I noticed a sign by the road. "Trout Pond" it said. I told myself it could be his introduction to fish-watching, a beginner's course. You really could see them, too. All the way from the parking lot. There were speckleds and rainbows leaping right out of the water. My son was thrilled.

But to get to the ponds we had to go through the fishing shack. There were rods there, and hooks. The bait was free. You only paid if you caught something. "Here," I said. "We put the food on these nice hooks so the fish can find it. See?"

I was going to pull out. I was. I just wanted to tease them to the surface. But I felt a tug, and, well, everything happened so fast. It was a rainbow, fourteen inches long. I had to stand on it on the dock, it thrashed around so much. My son was terrified. He screamed and cried and wouldn't go near the thing again until it was headless and wrapped in a plastic bag. Even then he asked me to put it in the trunk till we got home.

We barbecued it.

I went back out on the air mattress again, the day after our trip to the trout farm, but I couldn't see a single fish. The water seemed murkier, and the weeds thicker. Then something moved deep in the shadows beneath me. It was a dark cloud of a thing, about the size of a log, with a rusted bit of silver, like a very old fishing lure, hanging like a pirate's earring near its snout. I thought I saw teeth, and suddenly I wished I were in my canoe. My toes were dangling off the end of the mattress. I pulled them in and lurched back to the dock to help look after my children.

We came home the next day. I never did patent my idea for a guidebook.

But before we left, I walked down to the point one last time, to the place where I used to cast my lure years ago. It was dusk, and the light was fading, but just before I turned to go I saw a flash of silver in the water. It was sort of a flick, like a shovel-sized tail waving goodbye . . . or maybe beckoning, daring me to step in a little closer. It was hard to tell which.

Farch

We never talked about the weather as kids. We played in the snow until the stripe of exposed skin between our mitts and our sleeves turned bright pink. When it turned red, we came inside.

But later, as every teenaged Canadian does, I took the first steps toward accepting the conversational mantle of responsibility for our climate and learned to complain.

It is a good, vigorous and cleansing thing to complain about the winter. It toughens the lungs and strengthens the resolve and unifies the population. Canadians have long known its value, and we have turned the cold complaint into a ritual dance, complete with stamping feet and clasping arms, articulated with curses and spitting and concluding with the final flourish, the disgusted throwing down of the toque. This ceremony has been performed in the vestibules and back porches of Canadian homes throughout the winter season for generations.

But now, as with many of our Canadian institutions, the cold complaint is under siege.

For one thing, it's come to my attention that the very arsenal of our complaining, our language, is horribly lacking.

Normally, when a population lives with a great deal of any one thing, it begins to distinguish between the various parts that make up that thing and, eventually, creates labels for those parts. Examples might be the Inuit having so many different words for snow, the French so many for wine and the Americans so many for theme parks, fundamentalist churches and unfair trade practices.

Conversely, if those smaller parts outgrow their usefulness, a population will then group them back together with a new, larger label. In the Canadian military, I'm told, the officers who travel from one foreign base to another have one word for all the bits of loose change of various currencies that collect in their pockets while they are abroad. In Greece they would be drachmas, in Germany, deutsche marks, and obviously of value. But once piled together in the officer's pockets, out of their native lands, in military parlance they become kaploofniks.[1] I think it's a great word. It sounds just like what it is—a clanky pile of stuff that is no longer particularly useful. Even a good word, however, is rarely a permanent fixture. If current trends continue, the number of countries willing to share their kaploofniks with the Canadian military will become small enough that the word itself might become as useless as the thing it describes.

This ebb and flow of language has always been so. Yet, in Canada, there are curious gaps, particularly where

---

[1] I don't know if this is spelled correctly. Katherine Barber told me about this word. She has a brother who works with the military. She's also editor-in-chief of the *Canadian Oxford Dictionary*, but even she couldn't be certain of the spelling. "Kaploofniks" isn't in the book. Perhaps the military should collect its kaploofniks and organize a campaign.

winter is involved. For example, we have no word for the wall of snow that is left behind when the snowplow passes by and turns a recently shovelled driveway into a patch of asphalt at the bottom of a dirty, leaden, grey canyon of sludge.[2] Canadians certainly have no trouble thinking of words to say when this happens, but most of them already have several definitions of their own.

We also have no word for what happens when a person walking on a narrow, snow-lined sidewalk meets another person coming in the opposite direction and both parties end up stepping this way and that, in unison, trying to get around the other. There. I'm no William Strunk, Jr.,[3] I

[2] I've since found out that this is technically not true. Katherine Barber, when she was telling me about the kaploofniks, also told me that there is a word for the driveway sludge canyon. It's a "windrow," and, unlike "kaploofniks," it *is* in the *Canadian Oxford*. The first definition is "A line of raked hay, sheaves, etc., laid out for drying by the wind," while the third is "A ridge of snow, gravel, etc., heaped along the side of a road by a snowplow, grader, etc." This is all very well, but rows of grain ready to be shipped off to market might, I'm assuming, generally be considered a good thing, especially to the farmer who owns the field. Not so the cascade of icy slop that leaves the motorist once again pinned into his driveway after hours of shovelling. "Windrow" is, in my opinion, entirely too polite-sounding for such an affront to dignity. What about something like "snowslag," "plowpile" or "pludge"? Or, seeing as the language establishment often codifies vocabulary long after it has become standard usage, perhaps we should just call it a "God-Damn-It-To-Hell-Son-Of-A-Bitch."

[3] Author of *The Elements of Style* (Macmillan), later edited by his former student at Cornell, E.B.White. It's a great book about writing well and efficiently. It is ninety-two pages long, including the index, and contains wonderfully short sentences like "Omit needless words," which does. My copy even has an efficient press quote from *The New York Times* (no mean feat) on the cover. "Buy it," it says, ". . . study it, enjoy it. It's as timeless as a book can be in our age of volubility." I had to look up that last word. It means "using too many words."

know, but that took thirty-four words and it happens almost daily. You'd think we'd be more efficient.

We also have no words to distinguish the various stages of winter, even though it takes up more than half of our lives. Summer, blessedly short, is divided into as many distinct chapters as a Dickens novel. There is "early summer," with its shoots of pale green, "mid summer," all full of buzzing life, the "dog days" of relentless heat, "late summer," with crisp front-porch evenings, and "Indian summer," too. We even have the word spring, which in this country lasts all of a weekend.

But winter, which begins right after the last piece of pumpkin pie is served at Thanksgiving and stays until the blackflies come out several biological lifetimes later, is simply referred to as winter—start, middle, middle, middle, middle, middle, middle and end.

I got into this on the radio early one Saturday last, er, well, last winter. It was near the end of February, and I had noticed that the days were getting longer and the sun was a lot warmer and the snow was better for snowmen and the air smelled a little bit greener and I realized there was no way to say all that except to say all that.

I asked if anyone had any better ideas for a name for the time of year. It took a while, but eventually, still in the middle, middle, middle of winter, we started getting some suggestions. One person offered "Halt," because it seems like it never will. Another—and this was clever, I thought, because winter was finally beginning to wane—suggested "Waneter."

And then came the winner—Farch. It begins approximately one lunar cycle after the solstice and lasts until the equinox, the caller explained. It has fifty-nine days, sometimes sixty, and on the twenty-ninth day of Farch you should have a Farch Party to shake all that farchiness out of your system.

I thought it was perfect. It *is* a farchy time of year. The late afternoons are farchy and the sun and the air are farchy and the snow is, too. It even says *farch, farch, farch* when you step on it.

But what I liked best about the word Farch was that it sounded cold and dull and bleak and grey, and yet was still fun to talk about.

I'd begun to worry. Even in the dead of drudging Farch, in recent years I have noticed a lack of ferocity in good old Canadian complaining. Given the demographics of an aging population, I think that means trouble.

Time was that aging and complaining went together like cold roast beef and gelatinous gravy. When our fore-parents complained about the weather, they worked at it. It was a duty. If they hadn't worked up enough bile to start yelling when they came in the back door, they went back outside and tried again.

But those days are gone. Canadians haven't just stopped complaining about the weather, we don't talk about it at all. The only form of weather conversation that is on the rise in late-twentieth-century Canada is about as far from our ancestral heritage of weather resistance as it could possibly be. It is on the Weather Network.

Five million Canadians watch the Weather Network every week. Of those, many don't stay tuned for long. They are simply checking in—Inuit looking to find out what kind of snow is going to fall, for example. But there are also people who really *watch* the Weather Network—not just flip by, but pull up a comfortable chair, pour a drink, turn on the tube and take it all in. And, I'm sorry to tell you, they are not the young ones.

We are all rolling into old age like a wheelchair on an entrance ramp to the Trans-Canada Highway, and instead of leading the charge with acrid invective and house-shaking vestibule-stomping, our elders are slumped glassy-eyed in the La-Z-Boy fumbling for the remote. And, are you ready for this? Not only does the Weather Network have a core of middle-aged to older viewers, it also has a peak viewing season, and it isn't spring, summer, fall or even early winter. It is Farch.

This is not good news for the tight-fisted, stand-out-in-the-cold school of civic control. The Weather Network's ratings don't soar because they show blizzards (even if they have to film them on Ellesmere Island). No, during Farch, the Weather Network shows scenes of Florida.

Florida. The place where you can buy Canadian daily newspapers on the corner. Canadians, it turns out, when they are not spending Farch watching Florida palms rustle in the breeze on the Weather Network, are running there: 12,200 Canadians leave this country every day through much of the Farch season, and most of them are not going to Norway.

To be fair, though, some are going to Cuba, which I can almost understand. Spite isn't usually a major factor in vacation planning, but I don't know too many Canadians that would give up a chance to take a swipe at Jesse Helms.

But that is not a solution to aging population demographics, civic unrest, sagging moral fibre or even international trade injustices, and I don't have one. I don't even have a subscription to the Weather Network.

But I've got an idea.

If we really want to keep everyone from running to Florida every Farch, all we have to do is build a bunch of narrow sidewalks across the border and force those 12,200 Canadians to do that thirty-three-word, back and forth thing all day long with the Americans coming up here to sell us their magazines and take all our fish.

It isn't a permanent solution, I know, but it might slow things down a bit. It would even make sure Jesse Helms left us alone. He wouldn't be able to squeeze past on most of those narrow sidewalks, anyway. But if he did, it wouldn't be hard to stop him. We'd just send in the Canadian military to ask him to hand over all his Cuban kaploofniks.

Playing Catch with Memory

One morning a few years ago I ended up talking baseball on the subway with a ninety-five-year-old man. His name was John McNally.[1] "I played at St. Mike's," he told me. "I was a pitcher. One time I played catch with Babe Ruth."

He had my attention.

"It was on Toronto Island," John said. "Babe was just going through town."

I asked John what year it was and without hesitating he said "Nineteen-seventeen." Then he got off the train.

I liked him. It was a great story. Not "I struck out Babe Ruth." Just "we played catch." I wanted to believe it. But John McNally's memory didn't seem very reliable. I had to tell him when we got to his subway stop. He'd told me which one he wanted and then forgotten it not two seconds later. I wasn't sure I could trust him on the details of one afternoon eighty years before.

I did some research.

When he was seven, Babe Ruth's parents abandoned him to a Catholic orphanage in Baltimore. After that, his

[1] This is not his real name.

only father figure was a Brother at the orphanage whose name was Mathias. Mathias came from Nova Scotia. Many people think that's why the Babe liked Canada so much. From what I found out, he came here quite a bit.

His first paying job as a ballplayer was with a minor-league team from Baltimore, the Greys. They were playing the Maple Leafs on Toronto Island when he hit his first professional home run. The locals around here like to say he pounded the ball so hard it landed in Lake Ontario, but he didn't. It was just a home run. At first I wondered if John McNally was dining out on that story, like so many others, but that home run was in 1914, three years before John claimed they met. And besides, Babe Ruth wasn't famous in 1914. There was no reason to remember much about him at that time. He was just a talented young player, and if he was known at all, it wasn't for his hitting yet, it was for his pitching.

It looks as though John McNally might have been a pretty good pitcher, too.

There are a lot of J. McNallys in the St. Michael's College yearbook for 1917, but only one of them got a write-up for his athletic abilities: "The best ball player in the class, and natural acrobat besides," it says. It gave his nickname: "Lefty."

The only thing I saw John McNally do with his hands on the subway was hold on, but he was using his left.

Babe Ruth was a southpaw too. A pretty good one. By 1917, he was playing for the Boston Red Sox. He had the lowest earned run average in the league and he was earning $10,000 a year—a fortune at the time. You wouldn't think he'd have needed any extra money. But throughout that time he still went barnstorming.

Barnstorming was standard practice for big-name players. The term comes from the biplane pilots of the day who would fly into the small towns in the Midwest, land in a cornfield and offer rides to the townsfolk for a fee. They'd stay in town for as long as there were paying passengers, then move on.

Ruth was offering rides too. Usually to the poor sods who claimed to be pitchers and hoped to get a fastball past him. I can only imagine how quickly the excitement would have rippled through town when the great young baseball sensation pulled in unannounced and challenged the locals to a game. Anyone who played ball in those places would have had a day job. The town probably had to shut down the bank and the general store and comb all the neighbouring farms just to get enough men together to form the teams. By then, on a summer afternoon, with the whole town at the ballpark anyway, what excuse would anyone have for not coming out to cheer?

Ruth barnstormed for most of his adult life, but he had to keep it quiet. It was expressly prohibited in most major-league contracts; the owners wanted all the money coming back to them.[2] Any local coverage of a visit by the great Babe Ruth would surely have made its way back to Boston. After that, any likelihood of further impromptu games in that town would have been whacked right out of the park. No reporter wanted to be considered a rat by his subscribers. So, finding a newspaper account of one of those games is almost impossible.

At least, it was for me. I searched every sports page from the summer of 1917. I spent four hours of a beautiful

---

[2] Imagine!

day in the basement of the reference library peering over microfiche copies of one yellowed sports page after another, and all I got was a headache. I was about ready to quit.

But then I tried to imagine John McNally, at seventeen years old, out for a walk on Toronto Island. There had to have been a lot worse places to be going to school in Toronto than St. Mike's. It certainly would have been better than being abandoned at an orphanage. John did have his worries when I met him—health and memory and the like—but I don't think it would be stretching too much to say he still had a bit of a sparkle in his eyes, and that sparkle would have been a bright light seventy-eight years earlier.

And, even if he was a worried seventeen-year-old, on a summer's day on the Island, a game of catch, a little of the Music of the Spheres, might have been just the thing.

So, if I think hard about that old man on the subway, clinging to the pole at the centre of the car and not knowing where he is, I think I can picture him at seventeen. He has his ball and glove with him, as he does everywhere he goes. He is throwing the ball in the air and catching it as he trots to the ballpark, hoping to snag a cheap seat in the bleachers or maybe even get in free. He throws a high one, and, in his haste, he sends it too far. He has to run to get it. He is running, now, with his eye on the ball, dodging people in his path, when he hears a voice...

"I got it, kid." And a glove on a hand the size of a bear paw reaches up, hauls that ball down, and young John McNally is standing face to face with Babe Ruth.

I kept looking.

When I finally saw the name, it practically jumped off the page. *The Globe*, Boston, Monday, June 25, 1917—"Babe Ruth Suspended."

He slugged an umpire because he didn't like a call. I'll admit, that made me wonder if he was really the kind of guy you'd want to be playing catch with if you were seventeen. What if you threw the ball too hard? What if he did? In my microfiche delirium, I'd built up that guy with the bear-paw hands to have a heart of gold and be full of pithy bits of folksy wisdom that would send our seventeen-year-old off on a straighter path, just like in the movies—the kind of encounter that a young man would later realize had changed his life for the better.

Looking at it now, though, I'd say that *if* John McNally really played catch with Babe Ruth in 1917, he was lucky if he got away with all his money, let alone his teeth.

The league suspended Ruth for ten days, which seems like mighty soft judgment for a full-blown case of assault of an official before a stadium full of people. The Boston *Globe* reports that he attended the games on Wednesday, June 26, and Thursday, June 27, but he sat, out of uniform, and watched from the stands. Then, for the whole weekend following, and right on into the middle of the next week, there's no mention of him in the papers at all, except for a note saying some guy in Chicago was publicly claiming that Ruth owed him $100 and hadn't paid up.

It sounds as though it might have been a good time to leave town. I'm sure a trip to the home country of his adopted father would have made him feel a little better about things, to return to the site of his first home run and see the townsfolk leave their jobs to run to the ballpark all because of him. It was an awfully nice time to be in Toronto. It was a holiday weekend. The Toronto *Telegram* reports perfect weather for the Dominion Day celebrations on Toronto Island, with a crowd of twelve thousand coming out to see the hometown team. It was a great game, too. The write-up took up the better part of a page.

But there was also a smaller game reported. The story was on the inside pages, with no real headline. It was nestled in a round-up of a few other local events. That game wasn't on the Island but at Riverdale Park. That's the only reason I noticed it. It's close to my house.

I decided I'd better try and talk with John McNally again, to see if he remembered anything else. I didn't know his address, but I looked for a J. McNally in the phone book somewhere in the area of that subway stop, and it turned out he lives in my neighbourhood, too. He didn't want to talk to me very much, though, when I called and came to his door. He was getting his dinner ready, and he seemed a little agitated, so I didn't bother him again.

Anyway, that report on the inside page doesn't say how many people were out at Riverdale Park that day in 1917, or, really, anything very specific about the game at all. It wasn't the kind of report you'd notice, even if you were looking. The only remarkable detail was that it wasn't very close. The winning team had an amazing pitcher. The writer called him "Babe."

Still Too Young to Get Dressed

There are moments of nakedness in any life. We are born naked. We might as well be naked when we die. And, in between, well, it all depends how grown-up we are.

In Canada, we have a tenuous relationship with our national nakedness. We know that a mature nation, like those in Europe, has as little trouble facing itself alone in front of the mirror as it does on the beach with its neighbours. And although they are much more puritanical, we admire the reckless Americans in New York and Los Angeles who unbuckle the clasp of the Bible Belt and swing it over their heads in rebellion. Those two extremes leave us, as usual, looking for trousers that fit—and, as usual, the drawers are empty.

Here, in the past few decades, our nakedness has swung from being a spontaneous and rash explosion of freedom (think of the "streakers" of the 1970s) to, amazingly, as recently as 1995, some lingering resistance in smaller centres to the idea of public breastfeeding. The only constant has been our unwavering interest in nakedness as long as it is on someone else. Canadians might whistle, sigh, cluck or whoop at a naked body, depending on the tenor of the time, but they always look.

And, in Ontario, they pretend they didn't.

At least, they did until December 1996. That's when the Ontario Court of Appeal ruled that Gwen Jacobs was not, in fact, guilty of anything remotely illegal or indecent by walking around the city of Guelph without a shirt, which she had, in fact, done, until someone called the cops and she was arrested.

She took the matter to court and won, and now Gwen—and, by extension, any other woman in any other part of the province at any time of day, night or year—can take a shirtless stroll whenever she pleases.

It is clear that the people of Ontario felt they probably should—as a progressive, world-class kind of place—be able to live with such a decision, and do so in a cool and comfortable fashion. And that was the case for the first six months. It was one thing for the court to decide what it thought we thought was right while we were all safely ensconced in the snows of December, but you should have seen the fuss once the first hot summer day arrived! The papers were full of editorials, there were arguments in every lunchroom, and hookers were told that if they were sunbathing for their own pleasure they were fine, but they weren't allowed to use their nakedness for advertising. Within a few days it became as plain as the breasts on your chest that Ontario could accept the idea of its citizens getting naked and becoming more comfortable with themselves, just so long as they didn't get too comfortable with each other.

Now in Vancouver, in the progressive West, it's another story. At least that's how it looks from here. I've been to Wreck Beach, the nude beach just down the hill from the University of British Columbia campus. Being naked on the beach was truly amazing. To be bathed in sunlight and prance over that warm sand into that lovely water felt fabulous. Completely free.

But even in the airy West, sooner or later, you have to come out of the water and find a place on the beach, among the other people. Naked people.

I was twenty-five. I was fifteen pounds lighter than I am now and still wore size 32 jeans—well, I could have . . . Anyway, the point is, for me, I figured I didn't look half bad starkers. But that didn't make a wink of difference. When it came to socializing and enjoying the company of my fellow naked Canadians, I was not comfortable. I'd been wearing clothes for easily 95 percent of my life, and for most of the other 5 percent I was in the bath.

I don't mean to discount the career nudists in the crowd. Some people there *were* comfortable. There were entire families with little children and grandparents, all tanned, all smiles, all relaxed and all naked. It was a wonderful sight to see. And that was okay, too. I didn't feel uneasy watching them. I don't know how they got that way, but they were happy and healthy and without the slightest inhibition, and I take off my hat to them, if not my pants.

But there were about fifteen of them and about four hundred of the rest of us: twenty-five-year-olds growing up as quickly as we could, lying on our stomachs and trying not to look at each other.

So, what to do?

Well, I think Wreck Beach must be close to the UBC School of Business, because it wasn't long before somebody figured out that four hundred people looking for something to take their minds off what else they'd taken off represented a sizeable opportunity. Wreck Beach on a nice day, if you haven't seen it, is the world's only naked shopping centre. There are people selling jewellery, carvings, pizza, beer, cigars that are just cigars and even T-shirts to wear home.

I opted for a slice of pizza, which was soggy, barely warm and not even big enough to offer any real coverage should I get suddenly shy.

But that wasn't the only problem. The guy was asking five bucks a slice, plus two bucks for a drink. I don't know if you've ever haggled with someone who's not wearing pants, but I felt more than a little compromised.

Then, after that humiliation, he gave me my change in quarters. Where was I supposed to put a pile of quarters? My hands were full of food and drink, and my other facilities, as much as I liked them, weren't much use when it came to carrying currency other than the family jewels.

So, if anyone is thinking Ontario's new topless laws are going to open the buttons to rampant nudity all over Canada—Anne of Green Gables all in the pink, chance encounters in Come-By-Chance, in the nude in Neepawa and miles of skin in Saskatoon—I wouldn't worry about it. Before we see naked commuters streaming out of the train stations every morning, we're going to have to evolve as a species in more ways than one.

Besides, how would we distinguish one middle manager from another without the power tie? Never mind. No, to me, the bottom line on public nudity in Canada is that we're just not ready for it. Topless? Fine, but it'll be a while before you see the shirts playing the pants in touch football. Mystique is hard enough to come by around here. What about the next G7 summit? Chrétien will *really* have to watch what he says when his mike is open. *Everyone* will be able to identify Bill Clinton. And anyone who says they feel an election coming on could get in real trouble.

All of which leaves me wondering exactly where Canada is right now in its quest for maturity. Which stage is it that has brought on all this premature nakedness, this bare-buff brouhaha? Are we a five-year-old who suddenly needs to close the bathroom door? A teenager lined up at the drive-in? You'd think we were past that by now, but this doesn't exactly feel like settled maturity, either.

I guess we'll get there eventually. And maybe, by then, fiscal maturity will have come our way, too. It's a nice thought, no matter how far-fetched it may seem today. Just imagine, Canada: an emotionally solid community of citizens, confident with our bodies, openly appreciative of our neighbours' beauty, sure of our place on the beach and not having to worry about where to put our change.

Clothes and the Man

It's been interesting to see some of the more traditional styles in men's clothing making a comeback. Along with the cigars and the martinis, pocket puffs are back, as well as tie clips, cuff links, collar pins and even the occasional fedora.

It isn't difficult to figure out why. Over the past thirty years, every aspect of a man's life—including his role in the workplace, the family and the community—has been swung around more times than the back seat on a roller coaster. It's no surprise a few of us lost our hats. Or that we're suddenly trying to get them back. Especially the kinds our fathers used to wear.

Leading a son onto the right path has always been tricky, no matter what you're wearing on your head. Now the difficulty has been compounded by the lack of a decent map. Sure, our fathers gave us one, but since it was printed the entire topography has been re-zoned.

All the while, the landscape of manhood, which used to be dotted with heroic poems of bravery and strength and unwavering definitions of what it means to be a man, has become strangely barren. No one seems to be quite sure what a man is now—except, at worst, if he's too much like what men used to be, he's a lout, and at best, if he's trying too hard to figure out what he ought to be, he's a bother.

Clothes give us something to tell our sons with relative certainty. "That's a fedora," we can say. "That's a tie. Those are cuff links, and that's a collar pin. Chances are the person wearing them is a man."

Not that the right kind of shoes are going to make you any more of a man, or, more precisely, a better man than you would otherwise be. Nor can they show you which steps will lead you anywhere better than where you are now. To be doing your best to be helpful and succeeding only in getting in the way is even more humiliating in a new pair of wingtips. No. Your clothes will not define your sex role. They will not do anything for you at all. Except, perhaps, provide you with a small task, a daily ritual, that is somehow intrinsically masculine and rewarding.

Tying a tie does require some taste and skill. It is satisfying when it works. Wearing a hat, for some, does require a certain amount of confidence. Even if only for the moment your hand reaches up to the shelf, putting it on is still a choice to be weighed. If you do decide to wear it, your posture and your purposeful stride will be sufficient reward.

It is unlikely, however, that any piece of clothing will bring on wisdom and integrity, a greater understanding of the man's place in the world or a balanced, mature and peaceful relationship. But if you are wearing a tie, with a tie clip, on a single needle, button-down cotton shirt, a three-season wool suit, new brogues and a fedora, at least no one will be able to call you a poorly dressed lout.

Banker's Friday Blues

I lost track of something important when my employer got around to providing me with direct deposit. That's the system that automatically blips my paycheque into my bank account every two weeks. Until then, I had to go to the cashier's window every second Thursday, get my cheque, take it to the bank and deposit it. Not that the task was that onerous. It was nice to be reminded how lucky I was to have work and a paycheque at all. But still, most of the time, being who I am, I'd forget to go to the bank that day and would have to sneak out on Friday afternoon, when the line-up for the teller was as long as bank president Matthew Barrett's shopping list.[1]

Over those years of Fridays, standing in line till my eyes glazed over, I sensed something changing. At first it was only the tellers. They still took care with the way they looked, but their clothes were becoming less formal. For

---

[1] Failing trust company
Sea-Doo
Langevin Block?
Lower profile
Hair gel
Portugal . . .

me, it was the same effect as meeting an old friend who'd shaved a moustache. Something was different but I couldn't quite put my finger on it.

Then the men stopped wearing suits, and I noticed. They were, thankfully, still wearing clothes, but, still, it was a shock. It was as though Fred MacMurray had turned up with a nose-ring. I made a few calls and found I was about the only one who was worried about it. All kinds of companies were encouraging employees to dress down. They call it Friday Wear.

Local legend has it that Friday Wear started with a United Way charity campaign at IBM. Employees gave two bucks to the pot and were rewarded with the right to wear jeans on Friday. It was so popular it stuck. But when I called IBM they told me they had long before decided to change the dress code. They said that with so much of the information sector working from home, or in small, casual office spaces, the suits were too formal. Customers were uncomfortable.

But that's not what the clothing people told me.

I talked to Debra. She's a buyer for one of the shirt manufacturers here in Toronto. She asked not to be more specifically identified than that because, regardless of their taste (or lack of it), executives still buy shirts. She said IBM had an image problem. You had Gates from Microsoft, in jeans and Nikes, making more money than most of Europe. You had the creative guys at Apple dressed in California Hip. So, who's the geek in the suit? When IBM saw that, according to Debra, they told their managers to relax, and fast.

Yikes. I know the man in a suit hasn't been likely to draw sobs of sympathy in the late twentieth century, but this is tough. Most of the businessmen of a certain age that I know still have racks of suits in their closets. It used to mean they were headed somewhere. Now it means they've missed the exit.

The trouble is, most male executives would probably rather go to an empowerment seminar, or be transferred to head of "Special Projects," than be told to start dressing creatively for work. Heck, most of them don't have anything in the closet to choose from, anyway. It's a suit, or the pants they'd wear to change the oil on the Buick.

So, if your banker is a man, and it's a Friday, and he seems a bit distracted, it could be that he's worrying about the Asian crisis. But it's just as likely that he's wondering whether his taupe Nehru jacket isn't just a little nervy with the cranberry pocket puff.

I don't know a lot about banking, but I don't think this is a good thing. Bankers are *supposed* to be boring, and they're supposed to like it, too. Sure, they can seem greedy and inhuman, but at least you know where you stand, even if it's over the trapdoor. When bankers are worrying about their clothes, they're not worrying about your money. And as nice as it is to see a little texture behind the desk, I'm not sure creativity is among the more desirable qualities in a banker. For a person who handles millions of dollars of other people's money all day, a vivid imagination could be something other than an asset.

Besides, if business would just treat this venture the way it does any other, and read the prospectus, it would soon be obvious that, given past performance, expecting any long-term gains at all from office fashion is imprudent, at best. There was that boom in tie width back in the 1970s, but who saw that coming? And besides, when it crashed, it crashed hard. Those senior managers who'd held out for so long were just beginning to catch on when, in what seemed like less than a pay period, the guys in the mailroom had all gone skinny. Bolo ties and narrow collars. The next time one of the board members showed up, he looked like he was wearing a flounder.

You'd think that would have been warning enough, but just a few years later there was downsizing going on at the very foundation of fashion stability. Remember Don Johnson—"Miami Vice" and the three-day stubble, T-shirts and linen jackets, and, are you ready—no socks?

No socks! These are guys' feet we're talking about, right? Two-hours-sitting-on-the-bus-after-work feet? Very sexy. Some people told me they really did see men going to work with no socks for a while back then, but I don't know. I called the McGregor sock company. They said business smelled just fine all through the '80s.

As far as I can tell, there's only one sudden turn in men's business fashion that ever came to any good. That one falls on Clark Gable's broad shoulders, and it happened in the 1934 movie *It Happened One Night*. Clark was tough. Clark was sexy. And, Clark didn't wear an undershirt. So, other men stopped wearing them, too. Instantly.

The undershirt companies just about lost theirs.

I still haven't seen the movie, but personally, I have always hated wearing an undershirt, and I'd like men to be able to take credit for its demise. But it wasn't men. It was women. Women bought 90 percent of the menswear in 1934, including the underwear. The men had nothing to do with it. Women wanted their men to be like Clark, and they didn't care how cold they were.

But that was years ago. Things have changed! Bankers don't even wear suits any more. And women? Well, they buy only 80 percent of the menswear now. That's right, guys. Any feeling of fashion empowerment is an illusion. At 20 percent, you're not even a controlling partner.

As far as Debra at the shirt company is concerned, that's the way things should be. "We can trust women," she told me. "They go through this all the time. Fashions come and go. Women know when to stand and when to run. But when men start thinking they can dress themselves, from the industry point of view, it's a disaster just waiting to happen."

I stopped by the bank on a Friday not long ago. There was an uneasy truce in place: suits on both sexes, the occasional cardigan, and no jeans. But off in the manager's office, I saw a young buck in a Chicago Bulls jacket, big baggy pants and a cap on backwards. He might have been a courier, but it was hard to tell. He looked awfully confident. A career fast-track suit, I wondered? It made me shudder.

So, personally, I'm just going to lie low a while longer. As far as I can tell, women have always sailed the storms of fashion better than we have. If they want to steer us through this one, too, that's fine with me. Besides, just between us, I've never really understood what taupe is, anyway.

Yarns of Former Glory

My dad gave me a great Christmas present a few years ago. I was so surprised when I ripped open the paper that my mouth flew open and no sound came out. There, in my hands, newly cleaned and beautiful, was his old hockey sweater.

The hockey sweater has been around for as long as I can remember. I've seen it in pictures that were taken before I was born—Dad wearing it shovelling snow, on canoe trips, or skiing on old wooden skis with grey metal bindings that look like medieval instruments. Not that my father is ancient; he's only sixty-eight. But, in the way a child lumps together the ages of all things older than himself, I always figured that sweater couldn't have been much younger than he was, and probably was older.

I've always loved it. I think the first time I borrowed it was when I came home from university for the holidays. It was cold. I needed a second sweater. After that, I never brought my own. That was seventeen years ago. I guess Dad finally noticed.

I don't want to give the impression that the sweater's only value is the nostalgia it brings out in me. It is a truly beautiful garment, just like the one Roch Carrier dreamed of all those years ago—the glorious *Bleu, Blanc et Rouge* of the Montreal Canadiens. It has a white collar with lace-up neck, cuffs that still grab your wrists tight enough for a holding penalty, and it's warm. It's 100 percent wool.

"That's worsted wool," Dad told me. "Longer fibres and finer yarns." He knows that stuff. He worked in fibres for years at a chemical company in Montreal called Canadian Industries Limited, or CIL. In fact, that's where he got the sweater.

You see, Dad never *played* hockey in it. I don't think Dad has ever played hockey, period. He's from Devon, in the south of England. They haven't played hockey there since the Thames froze in 1142, and, like I said, he's only sixty-eight.

He was a huge fan, though. We spent many a Saturday night watching the Habs and listening to Danny Gallivan ("Laflooer steps gingerly over the blueline . . .") call the game. Mom sat in the rocking chair, I sat on the piano bench, and Dad lay on the floor. That was his favourite spot in front of the TV. The carpet was a polypropylene and triacetate blend. "It wore like iron," Dad said, "nice and hefty." It was perfect for drifting from rapt attention to the dead of sleep without having to move.

That was the pattern, too, with just about everything from "Wayne and Shuster" to "Truth or Consequences." There was something about the hum of the picture tube warming up. The set would click on and, almost immediately, Dad would click off. But not when the Habs were on. For them, he'd stay up right till the third star was called.

But considering he was such a fan, the story of how he came to have the sweater seemed strangely dull. He'd always said it just turned up in the office one day at CIL and stayed around so long that he finally asked if anybody else wanted it. No one did.

That was what I remembered hearing, anyway. And it's funny, but it never occurred to me to ask why a worsted wool Montreal Canadiens hockey jersey would have been lying around the fibres office of a chemical company in Montreal.

Until a few days after he gave it to me that Christmas. The answer hit me like a Bob Gainey hip-check.

In 1957, the Canadiens were having trouble with their jerseys. They'd been designed years earlier for older rinks and outdoor play. But in the Montreal Forum, with the grill downstairs firing burgers like slapshots and hotdogs almost as steamed as the fans, those worsted wool sweaters were just too hot. The players were boiling.

So, the front office, swept up in the space-age notions of the time, considered an alternative jersey made of the miraculous new fibres being developed in the houses of industry. Why, they asked themselves, should the greatest hockey team on the planet, possibly the universe, content itself with overly warm jerseys made from the greasy hair of mere animals? Faced with the obvious decision, they commissioned the crack team of professionals in the fibres division of the giant chemical company CIL, a dynasty in its own right, to make a lighter, stronger, better and more modern jersey out of the best man-made fibres money could buy.

To make sure the fibres folks got it just right, they sent along one of the old, original wool jerseys for the company to copy. That original was this sweater. My sweater. It wasn't just an Eaton's catalogue knockoff, like all the other millions of jerseys I'd seen, like Andy Roy's cotton jersey that I coveted so dearly every day after school in the park throughout the winters of my eighth, ninth and tenth years of life. No. This was *the real thing*. If it hadn't gone to the offices of CIL, it would have gone to the very centre of the hockey universe—the smelly, dirty, history-filled, champagne-soaked dressing rooms in the lower levels of the old Montreal Forum—to be worn not by a chemical company fibres man, or his hockey-mad son, but by one of *Les Glorieux* themselves, the mighty Montreal Canadiens!

Good Lord! Why hadn't he told me that earlier? I'd been schlumping around the cottage in the thing for seventeen years! I probably wore it to change the cat box! That year, 1957, fell right in the middle of the greatest hockey dynasty of them all. Five consecutive Stanley Cups. The names of the players on those teams are the very wallpaper of the Hall of Fame. The fierce and fiery Maurice "Rocket" Richard! His deft and determined younger brother Henri, the "Pocket Rocket." Jacques Plante. Dickie Moore. And the man who made the position of hockey team captain more elegant, important and respectable than any of the political appointments he would later be offered and would gracefully eschew, the greatest gentleman ever to lace up skates, Jean "Le Gros Bill" Béliveau. The long, fine, worsted yarns of that sweater are the fabric of this country's hockey history.

I wore the sweater every day for a week after learning that. Had fate not intervened, I told myself, any one of those great names might have worn it, and now I was walking in the very shadow of their steps.

I met Jean Béliveau not long ago for a radio interview,

and, if you would, please allow me a few lines here to say that, although certain aspects of these paragraphs may be justifiably discounted as the mad ravings of a former child, the above description of Jean Béliveau is in no way an exaggeration. The man is charm, elegance and integrity itself. He has, in fact, to date, gracefully declined two Senate appointments and the position of Governor General, offered personally by the Prime Minister. He was voted to the position of team captain by his peers, and, as such, was leader of the team for ten years, four of which ended with Stanley Cup championships. His charities have raised millions. His record remains, after almost fifty years in public life, without blemish.

Even more impressive to me than all of that, though, was the honest attention he gave to me and to everyone he met in his brief visit to the CBC. A fan asked for an autograph while M. Béliveau was on his way out. I could only guess at how many times he has been asked. I wouldn't have blamed him for at least showing some impatience or indifference. But he stopped and talked. He wrote his name clearly and respectfully and, for those few seconds, focused solely on the delighted fan, who left the encounter at least three feet off the ground.

But after meeting him, and witnessing his grace and charisma first-hand, I had to honestly face the cruel fact that Jean Béliveau could never have worn my sweater, even if it had continued on its way to the Forum that day in 1957 instead of being rerouted to CIL. Not that the sweater has the stain of scandal on it, or that it is at all below the high standards of the great man. It's just too small. Jean Béliveau is at least six-foot three, with shoulders as wide as a workbench. My sweater is only a "Large."

I still think it deserves a little respect, though. It gave up a career in professional sports, a spot in the starting line-up on a winning team. And for what? Shovelling snow and changing the cat box. Okay, it had a nice family life and travelled a little bit. And, to be fair, it wasn't there for the Stanley Cup, but it wasn't pummelled senseless by Gordie Howe and tossed blood-caked into the laundry, either. You hear stories about professional athletic garments that make it to the big bench only to end up sidelined with a pulled thread. My sweater was spared that fate. Still, folded up with the civilian winter clothes in my basement now, well, I'm not sure if a sweater that warm could ever experience regret, but I wouldn't blame it if it did.

I tried to find out what happened to the modern, space-age jerseys that were destined to bump the steady and sweaty worsted wools from the line-up, but it doesn't look as if they ever made it out of training camp. No one in the Habs' front office could find any records of the deal with CIL at all. Dickie Moore had a vague memory of some synthetic-fibre sweaters, but it wasn't very flattering. "The ones with polyester?" he said. "They didn't last long. We smelled bad enough as it was."

I can't say I blame old Dickie for being blunt. I'm no fan of the plastic-bag-as-shirt school of haberdashery either. But I'm reluctant to be too hard on old Poly. We all make compromises. It wasn't worsted wool that put the mutton on the table at our house. Wool was the competition. If we were warm at night in our home, it wasn't because of anything remotely natural or wholesome; it was because of polyester. Tons and tons and tons and tons and tons of polyester. Dad worked with the stuff, for CIL and later for its competitors, for twenty-four years, all told. If his employers didn't sell it to the hockey teams, they sold it to just about everyone else, and then some.

Besides, fashion being what it is, all those shiny, stifling polyester shirts are back now. Kids are wearing them, proudly, even. It doesn't seem possible that they've already been gone long enough to be brought back in the name of nostalgia, but it *has* been forty years.

It's hard to believe. On the one hand, my part of that time feels as if it has gone by in a sneeze. But, on the other, look at what's happened. The mill that made the sweater is closed. CIL abandoned the idea of a polyester hockey jersey. Soon after that they sold the fibres division, and after that just about everyone, especially the provincial government, abandoned Montreal. The old Forum is closed. Danny Gallivan is dead. The National Hockey League has gone from six teams to three thousand, and now the president of the league is an American. And, as I write this, our country is still reeling from the shocking news that our best hockey players—not the best amateur players but a team made up of the very best Canadian-born players alive today—failed to win a medal, any medal, at the 1998 Winter Olympic Games.

I could blame that on the fact that their jerseys are made of some ridiculous fibre that could double as a boat lacquer, but I don't think that is really a problem any more.

I wasn't alive in 1957, but it seems to me that it might have been a good time to be in Montreal. It's easy to picture bustling, snow-laden streets, joyous hockey fans, drunk with the dreams of bright times ahead. I can feel some of that when I put on the sweater. It makes me think of a bar in Montreal I used to like. It was a hangout for some of the music students at McGill—Henri "The Pocket Rocket" Richard's brasserie, on Park Avenue. We'd go and enjoy the surly service and the spectacular pork chops under the watchful eyes of the stars of *Les Glorieux*, photographed in black and white and hung on every available inch of wall space.

Montreal was already suffering then, but you never would have known it inside Henri's. The place was booming. When I moved away, Henri was expanding. He was building an outdoor patio called "La Patinoire." It had blue and red lines painted onto an ice-white floor, and the railing was made of hockey sticks.

Jean Béliveau told me that Henri sold the business a few years back and moved to Florida, but who knows? Maybe the place is still there. On a nice spring day, it was a great place to sit and watch the city roll by. I could wear the sweater, and meet my dad there. Jean Béliveau still lives in Montreal. It's possible, if we sat out on the patio, near the blueline, he might just happen by. I could ask for his autograph and say it's for my dad, the wide-awake hockey fan, and enjoy the moment as Jean signed his name, slowly and carefully and full of respect.

It's a long shot, I know, and it would only be a few seconds, but, when forty years can fly by like a slapshot from the point, leaving, as their only trace, a few strands of worsted wool, then really, what else have we got?

Both Sides Now

The twentieth century has not been a good time for answers. Questions have done all right—as well as ever, really, or better. What is the purpose of human life? What is happiness? Why do we feel the urge to know these things in the first place? My feeling is, we used to think we knew. The purpose of life was to get through it. Happiness was an accident. And, if you were asking why you felt the urge to ask those things, you had too much time on your hands.

But here in the prosperous *fin de siècle*, one of the main purposes of life seems to be to acquire so much wealth that you'll have nothing to do but wonder why you're still not happy. And why you want to know. And why you still don't have any answers.

That's the scary one for me. It's been shown over and over again that people become more conservative as they age. They start demanding answers. They won't settle, any more, for that open-ended stuff they used to happily wrestle with in university. To hell with some prof who says that happiness is "Whatever individual political actors take it to be."[1] As the vast and demanding tidal

---

[1] Thank you, Mark Kingwell, for a short answer to this question. If

wave of humanity that is the baby boom enters its senior years, and expects to get answers as quickly as it got bell-bottoms, a new stereo, sex, a house, better schools for its kids, a Dalmatian and a diversified portfolio, it is going to get ugly.

Be that as it may, I'm sorry to say that I don't have any answers to those big questions. I can, however, offer two predictions that might be of comfort in the increasingly nebulous and intolerant years to come. The first is that, before the dawn of the next century, there will be a fervent return to binary logic, and the second is that, along with that return, there will be hats.

I used to have a hat. It was a tan fedora with a black band and a green feather. I bought it years ago, just before Christmas, in New Haven, Connecticut. I wasn't planning on buying a hat that day, but I was out for a walk downtown and I was feeling a little blue. I was graduating that spring, and life was getting complicated. I had this prof who was in the habit of asking us giant, unanswerable questions and telling us that we had to answer them for ourselves. I went for a walk, looking for answers, and I found Delmonico the Hatter.

That's what the store was called, but that's who sold me the hat, too. Joe Delmonico, the hatter. He'd been making and selling hats there since 1926, when he'd started helping his dad in the shop.

Now, I'd heard what they say about hatters. But Joe didn't seem trimmed at the brim at all to me. All I did was

---

you want Mark's long answer, which is totally satisfying and might even make you happy, read his book *Better Living: In Pursuit of Happiness From Plato To Prozac* (Toronto: Viking, 1998).

ask "How much for a hat?" and in about thirty seconds Joe had sized me up, picked the perfect hat out of about three hundred lying around the store and placed it on my head with the authority of an experienced professional.

"That," Joe said, "is a great hat."

He was right. I loved it. And, after Christmas break was over and I wore it to school, I found Joe's assessment of my hat to be not only accurate but a universal truth. "Great," as it turned out, was, in fact, the correct way to appreciate a hat. My prof of the giant questions even said so. "That's a great hat," he said, when I walked into class. And to me that was good, as opposed to bad.

I didn't know it at the time, but Joe Delmonico, when he sold me that hat, had opened the door to the strength and clarity of binary logic. Nobody uses indecisive adjectives like "sensible" or "appropriate" to describe a hat. No. Some hats you put on your head to serve a sensible function, such as repelling rain or ultraviolet rays, but when people talk about hat fashion, there are only two choices: "great" or "stupid." It's "That's a great hat!" or "Why are you wearing that stupid hat?" There's no middle ground.[2]

---

[2] This was never more evident than when, a few years ago, our prime minister, Jean Chrétien, took matters into his own hands when confronted by an angry protester wearing a floppy, hemp-like number with big drooping earflaps. Chrétien grabbed the man by the neck and, with teeth bared, shook him silly. Naturally, the press was on hand, and photographs of the incident were widely disseminated. But, though our own prime minister had been caught attempting to impose the death penalty by manual strangulation for the mere crime of disagreement, there was remarkably little fuss. Most Canadians, it seems, considered the protester the guilty party. "In a stupid hat like that?" the common sentiment went. "The guy deserved it."

It sure made things easier for me. I'd be out shopping with my roommate, Kevin. "White asparagus, Kev," I'd mention in the supermarket before dinner. "Four bucks a bunch, is that good?"

"No," he'd say, looking at his empty wallet. "That's bad."

It worked for music, too. Duke was good. Hank Snow was bad. Barry White was so bad he was good, and James Brown was terrible, but in a good way.

Of course, Kevin and I were hardly the first to discover the joys of this kind of thinking. Binary logic has always been with us, except when it wasn't. And sometimes it's been less than good, which, given the basics of the system, leaves only one alternative.

Joseph McCarthy comes to mind—are you now or have you ever been, or not? There were the emperors in the Roman Colosseum, with those condemning thumbs deciding who'd get to go out for pizza after the game and who'd be sliced up for the lions. And how about the Spanish Inquisition? Talk about inflexible! And what *is* the common thread among those three? An ill-fitting fedora, crowns of olive branches and mitres the size of the hedges in old Seville. Right. Stupid hats.

Now, on the other hand (there are two, after all), let me point out that binary logic needn't always result in crimes against humanity. There are subtler examples of its power. For example, in the spring of 1997 an intellectual giant named Garry Kasparov was engaged in a chess match with an opponent that was as binary as they come. Chess might be a complicated and subtle game of strategy with thousands of mathematical options, but Deep Blue, an oversized toggle switch in a filing cabinet, otherwise known as a supercomputer, was the party that eventually won the day. That's won, as opposed to lost. No surprise, really, when you think about which player was built exclusively on ones and zeroes.

There is something to learn from that. Deep Blue never asked itself any of the larger questions. It just made each little binary choice, one at a time—one or zero, one or zero, one or zero—and soon the bigger answers became clear. What was its purpose? To beat Garry Kasparov. What was happiness? Beating Garry Kasparov. Deep Blue didn't ask the next question, about why it needed to ask those things. It didn't *need* to ask. As it always is with binary logic, the course was pass/fail. Deep Blue already had two out of three.

I don't mean to imply that we should limit our questions to the narrow focus of a Deep Blue. For one thing, our purpose in life *isn't* to beat Garry Kasparov in a chess match (even though that might make us happy). But while we are figuring out what our life's purpose is, there are some small binary decisions we can make that produce results. Is this hat great, or stupid? Should I wear it, or not? And even the hard one: Why am I asking these questions? Easy. It's raining.

Maybe Kasparov should have been wearing a hat.

That's why I think hats are going to be making a comeback in the coming years. We are entering a time in which clear, irrefutable answers, no matter how tiny, will gain tremendous currency. With the raging, aging, answer-hungry boomers, and the uncertainty brought on by the turning over of the fourth digit on the calendar (from a one and some zeroes to a two and some zeroes—ooh!) every yes-man, evangelist and motivational speaker in sight will be throwing up half-baked truths like stetsons at the rodeo.

It's bad enough every time there's an election. How many times can we be told that we need to get back to the basics, stand up for what is right and start using a little common sense, when, in fact, we would be a lot better off staying where we are, sitting down and shutting up? Why is it that we think *anyone*, let alone a politician, can suddenly come up with real answers (that just happen to fit into a seven-second news clip) just because it's been four and a half years since the last time anybody asked?

This problem, too, has been with us always. Whenever there are political choices to make, the middle ground disappears and our choices are Left or Right, giving the entirely misinformed impression that one is different from the other. These days the Left acts so much like the Right that the Right is left to leftovers. It's always the same with politicians, anyway. They throw their hats into the ring and knock at your door, hat in hand. But at the drop of a hat, it becomes clear they were just talking through their hats.

Hang on to your hats, folks. It's easy to see why the public has so little patience left.

Right?

I wish I'd hung on to my hat. I lost it about two years after that Christmas walk down to Delmonico's. I left it in the overhead compartment of a commuter plane bound for Toronto from LaGuardia. There were ninety-seven businessmen in suits, and me, a trombonist, with a hat. I guess my hat made one of those clear-cut choices it was so good at, and, like Kasparov, I lost.

But I'm thinking I should find another one.

Clothes and the Man

I called Delmonico the Hatter the other day, and Joe answered. He's still there. It's been seventy-two years in the shop now for Joe, and ninety since his dad started the business.

Joe still makes the hats. They're still rabbit-fur felt. When I told him I'd lost my last one he said they'd make me a new one.

"Will it break my bank account?" I asked.

"No," Joe said.

"Will it be great?"

"Yes," he said, and he told me he could have it done in a week.

I considered asking him about the purpose of human life, and about the nature of happiness, and why I feel the urge to know these things in the first place, but Joe sounded busy. I could hear the clanking of machinery in the background, continuously chugging out decisions. Great or stupid? On or off? Who knows, maybe even left or right; right or wrong, and Queen or Rook?

I decided I'd better let him get back to work.

"Thanks, Joe," I said. "Hat's off."

Ties

Men's fashion spoke to me one morning a few years ago. I just happened to glance behind me on the subway stairs. There was a column of men in suits. Their jackets were open and their ties were swaying in unison like swords, marching to war, grey and menacing, without a single splash of colour. They weren't in league in any way, as far as I know, except for their gait and their choice of tie, but I thought it might be worth looking into.

I called a neckwear specialist in the garment district here in Toronto. I talked to Hi. He, Hi, said this tie uniformity was just a backlash against the novelty neckwear we were seeing in the early 1990s—Mickey and Goofy, GI Joe combat scenes, that sort of thing. But another neckwear source said it was a larger issue. "It goes back to the big spending days of the '80s," he told me. "Then, a man wanted a tie that said 'Hey! Look at me!' Now all it's got to say is 'Look, I'm just doing my job. Leave me alone, will ya?' "

That's definitely the message I got from that legion of greys on the subway. As depressing as that was, I was kind of excited to know that it actually worked. I have always thought that men communicate with their ties. We certainly don't do it very much with any other element of our standard business attire. The blue suit instead of the brown or the double-breasted instead of the single are not exactly enough to let the world know very much about a man beyond "I don't want to talk about it."

When it comes to ties, however, men have a history of communication that would make Robert Bly pound his drum. While the rest of a man's wardrobe has long been about as private and untouchable as his fountain pen, the tie has always been open for business. For a while there, in the heady days of postwar optimism, ties were trading so fast they made stocks want to pull up their socks. Thousands of American businessmen became swept up in the fad of tie-swapping. At its lowest level, tie-swapping was simply fuelled by a man's desire to be rid of a Father's Day present that didn't suit his suit. But it was also male communication at its most spontaneous. Men would see a tie they liked on a colleague and, right then and there, on the street corner or in the boardroom, loosen the knot and make the switch.

The pitchman of the tie-swapping craze was a man named William Horsley. By 1948 he alone had made more than 500 trades, often with perfect strangers. There were tie-swapping clubs, one of which boasted 3,500 members, and trades at the rate of 34,000 per year. Clothing stores got in on the act, too, offering trade-ins in the shop, as long as the discarded tie could be displayed for ridicule on the premises. And, at the height of their humanistic generosity, tie-swappers collected ties and sent them to postwar Europe as part of the relief effort.

Makes you wonder just how uncommunicative men really were back then, let alone how big their closets were.

Every one of those tie-guys was choosing to make a particular statement when he got dressed each day, even though he might choose to swap his personal message for someone else's during the morning coffee break. It might only have taken him twenty seconds in the dark that morning, rooting through the laundry to settle for dirty socks as he chewed the last of his porridge, but still, with men and clothes, a decision is a decision, and ties are one of them. Actually, they are two of them, because once the tie is chosen, it has to be tied.

I still remember learning how to tie a tie. The basic tie-tying lesson is always in the bathroom. That's the only place with a mirror that will do. And you have to use a mirror, or everything's backwards. I remember Dad, over my right shoulder, peering at my neck. Once around, then under and up, down through the loop, line it up snug... Oops! small end's down to your fly. Let's try that again.

That knot is called the four-in-hand. It's named after the way a coach driver held the reins for two horses with one hand, presumably so he could fix his tie with the other. Men have used the four-in-hand knot to express themselves since the Industrial Revolution, when fathers left home for work. Junior couldn't learn how to be a man by following the plow in the field any more. He already knew how to wear pants. So what else was there? He had to learn how to tie a tie.

The only other mainstream knot choice these days is the Windsor, named for the Duke, who had no trouble fussing over clothing. With so much time and money and all of that nasty monarch business out of the way, what better activity to occupy the morning than working on the perfect knot? The Windsor *is* the perfect knot, too. It is at once symmetrical and subdued, bold and authoritative. It also takes a long time to get it right. Perhaps the D of W learned it from his father, in what we can only assume was a very large bathroom. In his dad's time, a guy needed a lot more than ten seconds in the bathroom before he ran out to church.

In 1828 there were at least thirty-five ways to tie your neckpiece. Honoré de Balzac even wrote books on the topic. One, called *L'art de mettre sa cravate*, was written under the name Baron L'Empese, which translates, roughly, to "Baron Stiff and Starchy." Not entirely a serious text, to be sure, but it was based on the kinds of things that men with little else to pull on their necks were worrying about at the time. It lists knots for seventeen- to twenty-five-year-olds, knots for sleeping and knots that were only for breakfasting and should never be worn in public. There were knots that caused apoplexy, too. Balzac tells you how to tie that one, and what to do when you collapse.

And there was even the Gordion knot. If you're up on your ancient haberdashery history, you'll know it was the one that was so complicated that, once it was on, it stayed on, and the only way to take it off was with a knife. Now *there's* a male fashion statement. It's not just a neckpiece, it's a pelt.

In fact, I do have one expired tie in my collection. It was my first bow tie. I wore it while playing a concert with the Boston University Symphony Orchestra. The piece was Prokofiev's Symphony no. 5—all kinds of big parts for the bass trombonist. It was the first concert of the year and, a few weeks before, I had found out that the men in the orchestra were required to wear tuxedos. Tuxedos. That we were mere students training for a profession that leaves most people too hungry to keep a shirt on their backs, let alone a tuxedo, was an irony that was apparently lost on the administration.

The only solution was a neighbourhood thrift store called Keezer's. They had racks of tuxedos only steps from the grave. But the bow ties were brand new, still in the plastic, and available in two distinct styles: pre-tied or authentic. What choice did I have? I was an artist.

The salesman, Mr. Keezer himself, showed me how to tie a bow tie. He was a pro. No bathroom mirror. I tried it myself with him watching, got it right, paid and left. I didn't think of it again until the night of the concert.

Our conductor was Roger Voisin, the great, former Principal Trumpet of the Boston Symphony Orchestra. He still had dazzling technique and a voice so nasal you could feel it in the back of your throat when he talked. If the violins weren't getting something right, he would sing it for them, using the original solfege (do, re, mi, etc.). If that didn't work, he'd ask one of the trumpet students to pass a horn up to the podium. It would be passed hand to hand through the woodwinds and violists up to the humiliated string player in question, and M. Voisin would then play the passage flawlessly, smile for our inevitable applause, pass the horn back, undo his fly and belt, re-tuck his shirt, do himself back up and away we'd go again.

Roger Voisin was also a stickler for discipline. Mistakes were fine if they were honest and the student was doing his best, but if there was the tiniest element of sloth involved, it was trouble, and tardiness was a sin of unforgivable proportions. If the concert was slated to start at eight, his baton would come down at eight o'clock, to the second, exactly as promised, and not one moment later.

I arrived at the hall early that night. I cleaned my instrument and warmed up. Then at ten minutes to eight, I put on my new tux. The tie goes on last.

It was three minutes to eight when I remembered I was going to have to tie my own bow tie, for only the second time, with Mr. Keezer's lesson rapidly receding in my memory. It never occurred to me, as I tried and tried again in the boys' bathroom, that since M. Voisin was in the almost daily habit of undoing his pants in front of seventy-five students just so he could straighten his shirttails, the sight of one slightly mis-tied bow tie in the back row of the orchestra was probably not going to bother him very much, while being late for the concert would almost surely result in capital punishment, with the chosen method being hanging from the podium by a bow tie at the first available musical break. Still, with panicked, fumbling fingers, I tied and retied and retied my new bow tie, never quite getting it right, with the seconds ticking ever closer to my certain demise.

I think it was about the tenth try that finally worked. The only thing that saved me was that, because the trombones sit in the back row of the orchestra, I was only four steps from the door at the rear of the stage. I took those four steps, saw M. Voisin raise his baton, took a breath, sat down in exact unison with his beat, so that my hind end landed on the chair at precisely the instant the piece began, and away we went.

If a man's ties can communicate, that bow tie still talks to me. I keep it in my trombone case, and years later it still says "AAARGHH!" loud and clear.

I've never forgotten how to tie a bow tie.

I even taught my father how to tie a bow tie. He had

just retired. It made me feel like an adult to be able to show him some of the skills I'd learned out there in the battlefields of life, where the conductors undo their pants and the tuxedos are all second-hand. But I didn't buy Dad's bow tie at Keezer's. I went to a stuffy men's store in downtown Toronto, which, as a seasoned bow-tie-tier, I could snicker at for its provincial snobbery. I bought a bright-red bow tie and a matching pocket puff—an apt expression, I thought, of my father's new position in life as a man of leisure.

I don't think he's worn it very often, and, the truth is, I knew that would happen before I bought it. But teaching him how to tie it just seemed like something I wanted to do.

We used the bathroom mirror, of course, my face over his shoulder. Fathers and sons aren't usually very good at saying the important things; I guess I was hoping the red bow tie might do the talking for me. I can still see our faces in the mirror. Two big smiles and a splash of colour.

Maybe, with men, that's as clear as a message can get.

Toe Rubbers

My thirty-fifth birthday hit me pretty hard. Of course, it wasn't as though I couldn't have seen it coming—I'd been thirty-four for 364 days at the time. Still, I managed to avoid the idea for most of the year. Until I was leaving for work one morning, and I looked at my feet.

Toe rubbers.

I'd had them for almost five years. I still remember buying them. It wasn't a big decision, I just found myself going more places in my dress shoes and not knowing where to put my boots. Toe rubbers were a practical solution. And for those first few years, even when I looked down and saw them on my feet, the whole thing seemed more like a lark than anything else. It was the same as wearing vintage clothing. It was nerd-hip. I was an artist. I was young. Then I wasn't an artist. Then I wasn't young. Then I was a balding thirty-five-year-old dressed just like his father on the way out the door to catch the train to work and—Oh, Lord! What happened?

I started to see a pattern in the times when I needed my toe rubbers: job interviews, church committee meetings. Never a beer bash or a pub crawl. And then I found myself, in my toe rubbers, in a real estate agent's office.

I left them there. Whether on purpose or not, I can't say. But I know that for the next few months I enjoyed a fleeting sense of freedom. I also had cold feet a lot of the time. But, in the end, clearly they never got cold enough. Within three months we'd bought our first house. On moving day, the real estate agent came over with a present: a bouquet of flowers and, in a plastic shopping bag, my toe rubbers.

That's when I gave in.

Wearing toe rubbers didn't mean my feet were always dry. Mine are kind of the sports coupe of toe rubbers—the low-slung loafer type that cover the back of the shoe and have about an inch of freeboard along the sides. Among their kind, they are stylish and sleek, if not all that functional. If I get caught in the average curbside slush pond, for example, my loafers are marinating all day.

It doesn't have to be that way. The style-versus-function debate has been raging in overshoes since the 1840s. That's when galoshes first gallumphed onto the fashion scene. Within just a few years there had arrived a dizzying array of choices: calf-high or slip-on, zippered or buckled. In the jazz age there were red rubbers, grey rubbers, two-tone rubber spats, slip-ons in the shape of wingtips and loafers. The Bata Shoe Museum here in Toronto even has a pair in tartan.

It all started with Charles Goodyear in 1839. The process he developed made natural rubber stable enough to be used in footwear. Not that it did him much good. Despite his enormous discovery, his finances never stabilized at all. He spent all his money protecting the patent and died $200,000 in debt, while a monstrous tire conglomerate, which would eventually feature a balding goof as its pitchman, prospered under poor Mr. Goodyear's very name. Trudging to work through the slush those last few days, what do you bet he had on his feet?

The funny thing is, he thought he was making footwear for women. In the beginning, almost all shoe rubbers were made for female feet. Men didn't have time for such foppery. They were working! But by the 1950s, the real question wasn't who wore the pants in the house—it was who wore the rubbers.

So far, around here anyway, that's me.

It's hard for me to believe now that it's been eight years since I trudged out of the Canadian Tire store in North Bay, Ontario, with vulcanized soles and a load on my shoulders. Eight years is probably a record for longevity. Toe rubbers are notorious for falling off. When I was a kid, Ste-Catherine Street in Montreal was littered with them.

Until the night of a hockey game.

It's in the old Montreal Forum that the toe rubber found its highest calling. It was a sort of celebratory confetti to heave onto the ice after a goal. The first time I went to a Canadiens game at the Forum, Frank Mahovlich scored his five-hundredth career goal. The ice looked like the Eaton's footwear department on a Saturday afternoon. They scooped them off with shovels.[1]

I see why now: these were middle-aged men, vulcanizing themselves with the virility of their lost youth at a hockey game. Naturally, when the time came for release,

---

[1] That's *Senator* Frank, now. Lord knows what they'll be heaving at "The Big 'M'" in the Upper Chamber in the years to come. Let's hope he's wearing rubbers.

what else would they cast off but the very symbol of their burden, the weight they dragged to work every day?

I'm told that in the old Forum the management used to leave the pile of expired rubbers on the sidewalk outside the loading dock after the game. It was a moment of brotherhood for the Montreal faithful to pick through the pile before they set out once again in the slush, back to their responsibilities and routines.

I don't know if that happens after the games in Montreal's new arena. I haven't been to a hockey game in Montreal for quite a while. Maybe I've been working too hard. I'll be forty in another couple of years. I don't feel the need to run from my toe rubbers any more, exactly, but still, an evening of abandon might be a healthy thing. I think I might be better, now, at facing the world, as long as I can step forward with confidence, without having to worry about losing my grip.

Milestones & Headstones

We Canadians are often told we are good at finding compromise. Most of the time it's a Canadian who is saying this, but we take pride in our achievement, nonetheless. At the table of international trade bargaining, over the endless conveyor belt of constitutional wrangling and even in our day-to-day lives, we live by the bland, steady light of compromise. It's our niche.

But there's an ugly side to compromise, too. For every deal brokered between the more outrageous and more fortunate than ourselves, there is a deal-maker who caved because it just wasn't worth fighting any more. What's more, "achievement" and "compromise" are natural enemies. Achievements are fleeting by nature. They also take lots of hard work, so we try to hang on to them. We cajole, we bargain, we tell ourselves we deserve to stay at the peak of achievement, enjoying the view, and yet, before we know it, we have slipped thousands of yards down into the valley of compromise. The joy of marriage is supported by the ugliness of divorce. The optimism of parenthood is shadowed by the appearance of unfortunate family traits.

In those terms, compromise doesn't bring the greatest good to the greatest number, it lowers all standards and leaves us mired in mediocrity. This is the basis for a national identity? When I have climbed the mountain, I don't want to be reminded that the only available direction is down. Especially when there *is* plenty more above—spectacular views and thrilling adventure—but I won't be seeing it because I'm just too old to climb any farther. I can call it compromise and, as a Canadian, boast about it, but it's nothing to be proud of. It's just the way it is. I'm stuck here, whether I like it or not.

But even being stuck isn't really the problem. The problem is accepting it. Living with the results of compromise is easy. The hard part is admitting to it. Even for a Canadian.

Personally, I'm hoping my feelings on this will change. I don't want to spend the rest of my days obsessing over how much nicer the view could be. I also don't want to worry about how much dingier it will be in a couple of decades when I'll be sitting even closer to the bottom of the hill, or, after that, when I'm in the back seat of the rest-home bus, parked outside the souvenir shop with a bumper sticker that says "I Climbed Mount Compromise, Almost."

I'm hoping that won't happen.

Because, all else aside, it *is* pretty nice up here. It's nice not to be worrying about falling. It's nice that, after all these years, I've found a comfortable spot I can tolerate for a while. It's nice to be able to look out and still see something worth looking at—the tops of a few trees, maybe, or some blue sky, a bird—and to be content with just that.

You could come on up and see for yourself, if you'd like. I know it's a bit of a climb, but do your best. Tell you what: I'll wait for you, and if you can't get this far, I'll come down a bit and meet you in the middle.

Here We Go

I'll tell you right now, none of the names I'll use in these next few pages are real. They're all friends or relatives, and I think I should respect their privacy. But they all did the same thing to make me want to write about them. They got married.

My wife and I were invited to six weddings a couple of summers ago. Two were on the same day. We had to split up. For the day.

There was Basil and Gwenneth in May, Jerold and Fern in June, Winthrop and Ralaida and Gandalf and Tilda both on the same day in July, Isis and Patrick in September and, on Thanksgiving weekend, Bindle and Fnan.

I told you I was going to change their names. And so I should. Once you get married, you might as well be somebody else. You aren't who you thought you were once that day is over, and neither is your mate. You might as well call yourselves Bindle and Fnan for all it matters. If you haven't yet found out for yourself, I'll tell you here: marriage is like a two-year-old in an elevator. It just keeps pushing buttons until the alarm goes off.

If you can find it in yourself to call a repair person, you're in luck.

You can't tell that to a pair of newlyweds, though. In fact, as the old joke goes, you can't tell them much. But you can try. That summer, in each of those six weddings, somebody tried.

The ceremonies ranged from a ten-minute walk-through before a justice of the peace to a Greek Orthodox celebration that lasted close to an hour, but there was one thing they all had in common. At a crucial point in the proceedings, after whatever trumpeting and fanfare did or didn't take place, somebody tried to tell the newlyweds what they were doing. In fact, in each wedding, the wording was remarkably similar, even in Greek. It was something like: "You are entering a relationship so profound it will change everything about the way you see the world."

I don't know if any of them really thought about it at the time.

I remember the minister saying that at our wedding. Now, who knows how much of our brains are actually listening at any given time? Sometimes I think there's a whole lot of unused real estate back there. If a musician can play a Tchaikovsky symphony for two thousand people, perfectly in time and tune with the other one hundred people on the stage, and still be thinking about what to get for dinner on the way home or whether all the wedding invitations have been sent, I would say there are a lot more things in Heaven and on Earth, *and* in the back of our cerebral cortexes, than are considered in most of our philosophies.

I do remember what my *conscious* mind was thinking

about. For six months my head had been a clutter of worries. Was the music going to be okay? Was I doing the right thing? Would I feel stupid in that ridiculous suit? Would I remember the ring? Was I out of my mind?

Going through a wedding is a great test of a relationship. The only thing more difficult, I've been told, is going through a divorce. But, at that moment, when that minister told me I was altering my life forever, all I remember thinking was something like, "Well, here we go."

Not jubilation. Not fear. Not even comprehension. Just "Here we go."

Now, don't get me wrong. I might complain to my friends now and then, I might storm and fume and rant, but I don't really think I would change any part of my married life, the better or the worse. Then it was "Here we go," and now it's pretty much either "Here we are," "There we went" or, in times of crisis, "Here we go again." We've been married for eight years, and, at this point, it seems to me we'll be "Here we go-ing" until we're gone.

I've talked with couples who have celebrated their fiftieth wedding anniversaries, and, from the stories and photographs, they don't really seem to be that different from the way they were on the big day at the altar, so many years before. Yes, grey hair has crept in, and a certain amount of vigour might have crept out, children and houses and jobs and pets and neighbours and friends and memories and even values might have come and gone, but the main difference from day 1 to day 18,262 (fifty years) in most surviving marriages, and marriage survivors, seems to be the transition from "Damn it! I hate it when he leaves his socks under the coffee table!" to "He leaves his socks under the coffee table." Indeed. By that point, she might, too.

And in many cases, especially if either of them leaves their socks under the coffee table on a daily basis, long before it happens 18,262 times, the phrase becomes "I *hated* it when . . ."[1] But I'd wager, even after the most acrimonious divorces, once the hate has subsided and the socks have all been pulled up and the lives involved have moved on, most former spouses, even if they admit it only to themselves, reach the point where the "I hated it . . ." part is eventually dropped too. We do end up accepting most things about each other, whether we like it or not.

I'll grant you, it can be awfully hard. Those couples at their fiftieth anniversary celebrations are almost always asked what their secret is, and the answer is almost always the same. They say something like "You have to work at it."

In the minds of most unmarried people and newlyweds, this brings forth the image of an older person happily engaged in some sort of hobby-like activity. A white-haired man in his workshop, for example, sanding a bird-house, or a grandmother knitting a sweater. Slow, methodical, but pleasing work.

Wrong.

Marriage is brutal. It stretches you further than you could have gone alone. It hurts you more than you knew you could hurt. It is harder and meaner and more ruthless than anyone who isn't married could ever imagine. But, even as I write this, and I'm conscious of reining in my

[1] That's 36,524 socks, after all. Enough is enough.

condemnation for fear of sounding bitter about the whole thing, I must say that I am not bitter. Not now, anyway. And even when I am, if I am honest about it, I must admit that there is something deep inside of me that takes satisfaction and finds order even in that. This, when you think of it, is the mark of a very well-designed system. It's peopled by individuals who subconsciously choose to put the system above themselves. And, after the worst of the worst, when the better hasn't shown up for weeks, the system has them saying and thinking that, even if they could choose again, they probably wouldn't change anything.

That's what I find myself saying, and, if I thought I could take any credit for my brilliant life choices in this regard, believe me, I would. But I'm not sure how much choosing I did to begin with. I've talked to other men about this. The ones I believe all say the same thing. It just happened. They met, they fell in love, the roller coaster climbed slowly up to the top of that first big hill, and then it was time to close their eyes and hang on.

Here we go.

Which is why I think wedding ceremonies are important. Of course it takes forever to decide whom to invite and whom not to invite and who can't sit next to whom and why. Of course it is farcical and humiliating. Getting two people to agree on anything is almost impossible. Getting two families to agree on anything *is* impossible. Trying to make sure such an event comes off at all is the lucky couple's first clue that what they are doing is far, far bigger than themselves.

That summer of the six weddings, I watched a guy who had barely finished high school marry into a family where everyone holds a university degree. I watched a woman who loves to talk marry a man who never puts more than three words together and talks about his feelings even less. I watched a truck driver who's been driving non-stop for fifteen years promise to stay put with a woman whose family has never moved farther than the other side of town.

Here we go.

The last wedding of that summer was one of the best afternoons of my life. The bride was the kid sister of one of my best buddies growing up. And the groom, let's call him Bernie, is about the best friend a person could have. He was forty when he married. We, his well-intentioned friends, had all been setting him up with disastrous blind dates for years. He liked most of the women we sent him out with, but, in his own words, "there were no bells ringing." At one point he said to me he thought maybe he would be single all of his life. He wasn't particularly happy about that prospect, he said, but he thought he should face the possibility. Then, just weeks later, he met the woman he did marry, and with whom, within a year, he fathered a child.

I don't know what made those bells finally ring for him. Maybe it was choice, maybe not. Maybe, when the priest told him what he was doing, Bernie did think consciously about it and understood. I don't know. But despite everything I've said about how difficult and draining marriage can be, when I sat in that church, beside the woman I married, and listened to my dear friend Bernie in front of all of us say "I take you to be my wife," I felt like throwing my head back and whooping at the top of my lungs. "Hurray!" I wanted to yell. "Hurray for life! Hurray for Bernie! Hurray!"

The oddsmakers have it that three of that summer's six marriages won't last. It's been two years now, for all of them, and, as far as I know, they're all still together. I hear that, after the first year, making it through to seven (2,556 days) is the next big test. We've made it through that one, and in the process I've learned enough that I'd never accept a wager on who else will make it there too, or beyond. But if any one of those newlyweds is ready yet to listen to what someone is saying to them, I can offer this: Keep that elevator service number handy. Don't change your names to Bindle and Fnan. And, when you get to the top of that first big hill, just hang on tight.

Are you ready?

Here we go.

The Big Awake

I took only one psychology course in my academic career, and that was seventeen years ago. About the only thing I remember about it is how often our teacher, a clinical psychologist, told us he was a clinical psychologist. I'm still not sure I believe him. Even so, with each new disorder presented in class, we, the students, would surreptitiously eye each other, looking for symptoms, wondering if the others were wondering all the same things about themselves, and whether our teacher, the clinical psychologist, had stopped wondering and actually knew.

I also remember one case study on sleep deprivation. The subject was a radio host. I don't know his name, but I can still see his face in the black-and-white photograph in our textbook. It must have been in the early 1960s, because he was wearing a wrinkled, small-collared white shirt, open at the neck, with a narrow tie loosened and all askew. He was at a desk in a studio, behind a microphone that looked like the grille on a pickup truck. There were bags the size of fenders under his eyes and he looked slightly incoherent. The picture was taken just before the end of the study. At the time, he had been awake for five and a half days.

That picture popped into my mind on November 2, 1994. I'm sure of the day, but the time is a little murky. It was dark, anyway, and everyone else in the house was asleep. I was downstairs in the living room, sitting in a rocking chair, and wishing I were in bed. There was an eight-day-old baby in my lap. It was my daughter.

She was in good health. Nice birth weight, thick, black hair and piercing eyes that reminded me so much of my mother that I had to look twice each time I saw her. It wasn't an easy labour for my wife, if there is such a thing, so I can't, in good conscience, say that everything was totally rosy. We also had a twenty-two-month-old son at the time, who was far from maintenance-free himself. And, on the first evening my daughter and wife came home from the hospital, I put a brand new carving knife right through the tip of my finger. The gash went down to the bone. We'd bought the knife from a door-to-door type who'd stressed how well the knife would hold its edge. He was right.

I can't honestly remember which finger got the treatment; the knife was so sharp that there is literally no scar. But there was blood, and that brought a fair amount of confusion. One minute I was the proud papa providing sustenance for his brood by carving the leftover roast, and the next I was in the emergency ward looking like an extra from the set of a Freddy Krueger movie, babbling to every available nurse, intern, doctor, patient and cleaner that I had to get back home as soon as I could to be with my new baby daughter. They were very good about it. It took only a few hours. When the doctor did finally see me, instead of stitches he sealed the wound with a kind of Krazy Glue that actually burned my exposed and bloody flesh back together as pungent little puffs of smoke rose up. I roared and scowled, at which point the doctor smiled and asked, "How long did you say your wife's labour was?"

Aside from all that, things with our new baby were fine, except that she didn't sleep very much. Well, no, she did. It just wasn't when we wanted her to. A pattern emerged after a few days. She seemed to like waking up just before we'd fallen asleep. I'm sure you know the feeling. I'd done all my pillow placing and blanket pulling and turning over and leg adjusting. The house was quiet. The air around my face was cool, and under the covers it was soft and warm.

Then there was a gurgle.

It's amazing how much noise a baby can make. I was at least twenty feet and two rooms away, and her gurgles sounded like drainage from an industrial septic tank. After that she would sneeze, squirm and snort, and then it was time for me to pull off those glorious covers, find my clammy slippers and go for a nice, cold, long, dark walk around the house.

I thanked myself at those times for having swallowed my pride and bought a nightshirt. It was a forest green, knee-length number from the Gap, an attempt at youthful sleepwear, an oxymoron if there ever was one. The true sleepwear of youth, I can now appreciate from the distance of a few years, is the kind that stays in the dresser drawer, in a heap on the floor beside the bed or, better still, wrapped in plastic and still in the store.

As captivated as I was by the *Playboy* magazines I'd sneak a look at in the barbershop when I was a kid (before I decided to go to a hairstylist's), I knew even then that something about them was fake. It wasn't the reconstituted

Barbie-like models; I was willing to believe they existed. My problem was Hugh Hefner spending all day in his pajamas. The man was supposed to be the very symbol of randy youth. Randy youth doesn't wear pajamas. It is so boiled up in the froth of flesh that it can hardly get dressed in the morning, let alone at night. And when there is a fire in the hotel and randy youth turns up on the sidewalk with its paramour, the both of them wrapped only in a bed sheet, they are smiled upon by age. Their nakedness is a good thing. Age, in its cotton or flannelette, or forest green nightshirt, pulls its drawstrings and happily remembers the day.

I wasn't thinking about any of that when I bought my pajamas. I knew within a short time I'd be spending a lot of my nights with a baby who would be looking to me for guidance, example and protection, and somehow, success in that role seemed less likely if I was going to be naked.

As it was, on that November night in 1994, I don't think my infant daughter cared either way. Besides, I was proud to be the one walking her around in the middle of the night. Suffering the insult of pajamas in addition to the injury of sleep deprivation was the least I could do. Or, more accurately, it seemed to be about all I could do.

Many fathers I know have struggled to find a way to make themselves useful in those early days. Of course, their efforts have to be considered in the context of their female partners, who are struggling so much with everything else that they don't have any energy left to struggle with their men over how useless they are being. But, useless or not, I'm a light sleeper. We all have our gifts, I suppose, and, as a parent, that is mine. One industrial-strength gurgle and I didn't stand a chance.

Unfortunately, in the slumber department, I think my daughter comes from my side of the family bed. During the day she'd sleep through a hurricane. I even dropped a saucepan lid right beside her once. She was asleep in the bassinet on the floor of the kitchen, while I struggled with a vat of beef stew at the stove. I'd leaned forward to smell the vapours, and had almost fallen asleep on a parsnip, when my hand slipped and knocked a lid from the counter. There was a great *clang!* and then a circular *wanga-wanga-wanga* that seemed to go on for centuries while the lid spun to a stop mere inches from her head, and she did nothing. She didn't budge. But once it was past midnight, the sound of our creaking floorboards would have her startled and wide-eyed and greeting the blinding blackness. And, once up, she was up for a while.

My *Concise Oxford Dictionary* defines sleep as "the bodily condition which normally recurs for several hours every night, in which the nervous system is inactive, the eyes are closed, the postural muscles are relaxed, and the consciousness is nearly suspended." Doesn't that sound delicious? Oh, to have been able to close my eyes and have my consciousness suspended, just for a few more minutes. It was the stuff of fantasy to merely let the eyelids down for a second. The touch of eyelash to eyelash. The subtle sinking of the shoulders. The gentle, even, rising and falling of the chest in blessed, peaceful, unfettered succession. Oh, oh, oh.

In recent months I have come across several attempts to quantify the extent of sleep deprivation in our society. The results vary, but not one of them is cause for optimism. For example, in 1998 the U.S. National Sleep Foundation published the results of a study which found that 32 percent of Americans are sleeping as little as six hours or less per night during the work week, and 64 percent are sleeping less than the recommended eight hours. But those numbers mean more than just a whole lot of grumpy mornings. They also found that 30 percent of men and 15 percent of women had fallen asleep at the wheel of a vehicle at least once in the previous year. In a 1997 survey quoted by the Sleep Foundation, sleeplessness cost American employers $18 billion in lost productivity, as well as increases in medical costs, absenteeism, accidents and hospitalizations.

Furthermore, you don't have to have napping employees to be concerned. Mary A. Carskadon, a sleep researcher and professor of psychiatry and human behaviour at E.P. Bradley Hospital in Providence, Rhode Island, says: "Sleep may play a major role in, among other things, regulating mood and emotion. Most studies done on sleep deprivation look at performance, ability to think and reaction time. But you can speculate about the other consequences on society: increased violence, increased divorce rates, and an increase in the homicide rate."

Yikes. If not getting to sleep doesn't kill you, some other sleepy brute will.

Even if we can escape the spectre of drowsy diseases, sleep-deprived divorces and dangerous driving, what about all the other half-awake sleepwalkers around us every day? In that winter of my sleep discontent, entire weeks went by without a single conscious thought on my part. People recalled for me conversations that I would swear had never happened. Items that I had bought, but had no memory of, would appear throughout the house. I paid bills, worked, made promises, agreements, commitments, changed diapers and, presumably, slept every now and then, for what seemed like a very long time, entirely on automatic pilot.

In my case, this is not so alarming. My work involves talking on the radio and writing stories. The worst thing I could have done was send a character out for a walk, and forget to bring him back. But what about the person who flies an airplane? Or operates heavy construction equipment? Or determines the distribution of layoff notices? Those people become parents too, and I'm not sure I'd want to be a character wandering around lost in their stories, thank you very much.

It has even been suggested to me that sleep deprivation is used as a tool by hospital administrators to encourage more effective decision-making among their interns. It's already hard enough to decide which patient gets to take the one remaining artificial life-support system, or whether the young, suicidal smoker deserves the transplanted heart more than the emotionally balanced senior citizen. Philosophers spend entire careers pondering such questions; an emergency room doctor can't really be expected to have any greater insight. But, if they have been awake for forty-eight hours, they also can't really be expected to be able to care any more. "To hell with ethics," you can well imagine them saying, "can I use that bed when this guy's done with it?"

And, should we survive this daily night-of-the-living-almost-dead-with-lack-of-sleep, there is little rest in sight. It would seem that the moment we finally reach the stage of life where we are getting a reasonable number of hours in dreamland, a reasonable number is no longer enough.

All through those years of midnight madness, what

kept me going was the knowledge that soon, when my children were older, I would be getting as much sleep as I needed. If you already have children that are beyond infancy, you know what is coming.

What happened? My children *are* older now. They *do* sleep through the night most of the time. Sometimes I even have to wake them up in the morning. No matter. Most of the time, I'm still tired. The idea of "enough sleep" remains as unlikely as pajamas on randy youth.

Most of the men I know who are over fifty and work hard during the day have a nasty habit of sitting down after a nice dinner with friends, starting into a stimulating conversation and promptly nodding into oblivion right there in the living room, chin anchored to sternum, head flopping about like a pillowcase in a windstorm. I know, to them, it seems only moments ago that they were awake and pacing all night with infants (if, in fact, they were), but, I'm sorry, there is nothing chivalrous about snoring for company over the liqueurs.

I wouldn't be saying anything about this here except that it is already happening to me. At this point, I have to be in a very warm room and have had at least a couple of glasses of wine with dinner, but still, I'm only thirty-seven. I'm guessing it's not going to get any better from here on. I'm also guessing, judging from other observations in the field, that whether I want to or not, before long I'll start lying down on the sofa after lunch, before dinner and in between, and, when company's over, if I haven't snored them all away with my after-dinner snoozing, I'll be standing up abruptly at ten o'clock, no matter what stage the party is at, purposefully slapping my thighs and saying, "Well . . . !" as many times as is necessary, until everyone goes home. Talk about suspended consciousness! I don't mind if my nervous system decides to become inactive, as long as it doesn't make me socially inactive at the same time.

How it is that our bodies require progressively more sleep than our daily lives can supply, no matter how much that is, is a question worth reading up on, as long as the appropriate texts are not too long and are written in the active voice. But don't stay up too late with the nightlight on, either. The next phase after the post-meal, age-precipitated sofa-snore is the unrequested internal wake-up call. Strangely, as the years progress, most people find that, no matter how wiped they were the evening before, come the next morning, they are up at dawn and can't get themselves back to sleep.

In fact, oddly enough, as the years progress, it seems to me that most people in their final decades end up with sleep patterns that are surprisingly similar to those I endured with my infant daughter in the first year of her life: wide-eyed midnights, blindingly early mornings, midday naps of unfathomable number and schedule, drowsy evenings and mealtimes, plagued with either insomnia or narcolepsy, whichever is the most inconvenient.

It's enough to make you want to lie down.

But, in truth, not all my sleepless nights have been unpleasant ones. I can only assume that will continue to be the case. During that first winter of my daughter's life, there were things about our midnight visits that I began to enjoy, once I was awake. If I was coherent enough, I'd read her a book, which was often delightful. *Treasure Island* comes to mind. She seemed to like it too.

We also watched a fair amount of TV, which at that

time of night usually consisted of several choices of action movies with fantastic explosions and excessive violence, something I probably wouldn't have indulged in, myself, under other circumstances. She seemed to like those, too. I suppose I might pay for that in a few years.

Mostly, though, we listened to music. Our tastes have drifted apart slightly since, but back then we were kindred musical spirits. Of course, crying being her sole verbal expression at the time, I could only tell which ones she wouldn't tolerate. But, like I said, we spent a lot of time down there in the dark, and before too long I was able to put together what I gather she felt was a passable play list. It had big orchestra pieces with lots of brass, like Bruckner and Mahler, folk singers from the '70s, early Miles Davis, the Thad Jones/Mel Lewis Jazz Orchestra and the occasional Led Zeppelin.

I've promised to put together a tape that she can listen to with her children.

I can't say exactly how many months those nighttime visits went on for. I only remember that sometime midway through the next summer I felt as though I was crawling out of some sort of unconscious state and could begin to try to participate in life again. But there is one night in the early days that stays clear in my memory. It was that night I started telling you about earlier: November 2, 1994.

We'd been in the rocking chair for an hour or so. I was rocking, she was listening. Then Miles finished his chorus, and off she went. I could have put her down. In that first five minutes of real sleep she would usually sleep through whatever noise it took to put her in her crib.

Blissfully suspended consciousness was only steps away. But the house was dark, there wasn't a soul outside, and I was holding an eight-day-old baby against my chest: my daughter. She was curled like a tiny mammal with her limbs all tucked in, the smell of her skin right beneath my nose, her entire ribcage fitting under one of my hands. I could feel her breathing.

I stayed there half an hour.

The creaking stairs didn't wake her that night. In my memory, she slept right through till morning, although I could easily be wrong about that. Except for that one moment, all memory was instantly erased the second I'd put her in her crib. I was out in seconds, and very, very happy.

Incidentally, that radio host I mentioned, the one in my psychology textbook who didn't sleep for five and a half days? As I remember, the study got a little ugly at the end. After the fourth day, he really lost it. He was on air live, too—talking with guests who weren't actually there, speaking gibberish for hours on end and, finally, losing touch with reality altogether.

I really don't remember much about that winter, and since my job was on a morning radio show, and I was waking up at about the same time my daughter often did, in the middle of the night, and playing a lot of that music she liked, too . . . well, it's hard to know exactly what went on. I wasn't fired, I know that much. I suppose I could go back and read the rest of that psychology textbook to see if it fills in any more of the blanks. I've still got the book somewhere. It's in a box with my Led Zeppelin records. I'd just need to get them all out, find a nice, soft chair to lean back in as I read, lots of warm blankets and a bunch of delightful dinner guests in the living room, and I'm sure I could learn all kinds of interesting things. There's nothing abnormal about that for a man of thirty-seven, is there?

Go Back, It's a Trap!

I found myself thinking of my friend Jeff not long ago. It was the end of a working day and I was walking through the park. It was spring. The grass had begun to turn green, and the sun, mercifully for a city in the northern hemisphere still using equal-sized day and nighttime hours, had not yet set for the day.

I remembered Jeff when I saw a teenaged couple necking on a park bench. Not that Jeff was necking on park benches much, at the time. At least, he hadn't told me about any necking *al fresco*, and if he had I would have known he was lying. First of all, he lives in Halifax, where winter lasts even longer than it does here in Ontario. Anyone who goes necking on park benches before June in Halifax is at risk either of hypothermia or of being washed out to Sable Island in the annual spring run-off that sweeps the downtown area of loose rubbish, discarded large appliances and necking teens.

But even if Jeff had lived in Aruba, he probably wouldn't have been managing much necking at all. Jeff and Joy, his wife, are the parents of twin girls. The girls are delightful, but they don't care about their parents' necking time. No.

I thought of Jeff when I saw the necking teens on that wonderfully bright spring evening, not because of any recent necking he had done, but because of something he had said to me years before.

It was while he and Joy were expecting. Their pregnancy was big news. Jeff and Joy had been together for years, through career changes, cross-country moves, several cars of what can only be kindly described as dubious reliability, not to mention a few dips and swoops on the marital roller coaster. They had resisted the idea of having children through all of it, and then some. It was pretty much the last minute of play on the procreational clock when they decided to run for the goal line, and then things took a while to get started. Everyone was thrilled when they announced they were pregnant, and none more than Jeff and Joy.

I know Jeff because we worked together for a few years in Halifax. We produced a radio show that was broadcast on what the CBC then called its Stereo Network between five and eight in the mornings on the weekend. One reviewer referred to it as "The Siberia of Radio." This judgment was, perhaps, overly harsh, but it didn't bother us. We had a great set-up: a big office with a big sound system, at the end of a long and narrow corridor. We played very loud and strange music all day long. I don't know how many managers, colleagues or even friends approached that door and then thought better of it, but we seemed to have lots of time to talk.

I had moved away by the time Jeff and Joy began their journey into parenthood, but by then our conversational patterns were set, and we still talked often by phone, that year especially. We talked about fatherhood, marriage, and, mostly, seeing as my own daughter had only just graduated to toddlerhood, we talked about babies.

There were three trimesters to our baby talk. The first was what you might expect: lots of high-speed babble, interspersed with heavily researched comparisons of crib construction, stroller design, shelving systems, and the environmental consequences of the various diaper options. There was also plenty of awestruck silence from Jeff on the other end of the line, with the occasional sparse word or two clearly being spoken through a grin.

Our second trimester of baby talk began the day Jeff told me they were expecting twins. There was still plenty of babble and awe in his conversation, but, more often than not, I could tell, the grin was gone. It's not that he was any less delighted at the prospect of two children than he had been at the prospect of one. It was that, what with the size of the idea of twin parenthood, of multiple procreation and of Joy, he was beginning to feel rather small.

By the time they have reached adulthood, most men have become used to the idea that they are rather large in the landscape of their own lives. This statement will have elicited eye-rolling from most female readers. I am merely trying to set the scene. Because, with expectant fatherhood, the male of the species, if he chooses to think about it, has little choice but to face the fact that his last biological contribution to the process was a microscopic tadpole, while his female partner in parenthood gradually becomes as large, and as vital, as the entire pond—in fact, a walking ecosystem. That most men, however, manage not to think about this is, while embarrassing to those men who do, still a tribute to the system. Nine months is the perfect gestation period for human beings. It's long enough for a guy to paint the nursery and build all kinds of ridiculous shelving systems without ever really absorbing his own insignificance, or what that colossal insignificance has gotten him into.

I guess Jeff was either more secure or more astute than most of us, because our conversations on this topic changed forever one morning, about two weeks before the twins' due date. "I've lost control," he told me. "I can see it happening and it's still too late. I used to feel that I was still making my own choices, but now, everything's changed. I've been enveloped. My thoughts, my money, my independence . . . it's all been sucked up into that, that . . . womb, and there's nothing I can do about it! I was walking through the park and I saw a couple nuzzling on a bench by the fountain. They were kissing and gazing into each other's eyes, all dreamy with love, and I couldn't stand it! I wanted to run up, shake them and say, 'Don't do it! Go back! It's a trap!'"

It makes me think of the business of pheromones busily sending their potent ready-for-sex messages. It's not the idea that our bodies are sending subconscious smell signals that I find disturbing, it's that they do it without asking. It *is* a trap, and pheromones are the bait.

It's one thing if you're a balding, nineteen-year-old skirt-chasing wag, actually interested in finding a mate, but what if you're not? What if you'd like to think you've outgrown that sort of thing? What if you're already married and happy, or trying to get over a break-up, or maybe just trying to get a little work done? Pheromones don't care. They don't care how many babies you have produced, or how little time or money or even interest you have in producing any more. They don't care that you've already stepped in the trap and have been successfully caught, and you are now living, in what might resemble a responsible fashion, with the consequences. They don't care how tired you are. Or how tired the object of your affection is. They don't even care *who* the object of your affection is.

In an enlightened society that promotes some form of civilization, or at least social conformity, pheromones are not part of some time-honoured regulatory system for healthy genetics, they're criminals. They don't care about marital fidelity, or child-support payments, or adequate life insurance. They're worse than us.

And, here's the scary part, they *are* us.

Is there anything or anyone else that you would trust if they started calling people you didn't know and setting up dates without asking you first? It makes you wonder what else is going on back there. If we're divided into parts that are on our side in this and parts that aren't—how do we know who is who? That nice smile we gave that woman on the elevator, where did that come from? Who thought of that funny line at the party? Who forgot the deodorant?

Of course, if I were a woman, the idea that there were parts of me I could trust and parts I couldn't might not seem so novel. I don't mean to say that women are any less unified in their emotions than men are, just perhaps a little more aware. After all, who buys most of the birth control in this country? A lot of women who don't want to get pregnant, that's who. There's nothing like the idea of seeing yourself turn into an ecosystem to cool your interest in microscopic tadpoles, or at least make you more aware of how many there are in the pond. Make no mistake—the pharmacies may call it "family planning," but deciding to not get pregnant is not simply a matter of planning. It is a struggle. Pheromones, hormones, backbones—they're all on the other side, and they are playing for keeps.

At universities, where there are lots of young people, and even more pheromones, and where nobody wants to get pregnant, they refer to the students as a group with the term "student body." It's not a very elegant use of language, I'll grant you. William Strunk, Jr., was supposed to have preferred "studentry." But for the purposes of this discussion it nicely wraps up the idea of a bunch of individual creatures, or impulses, all in the same place, all affected by the others' actions, trying to do something together. There is the student body, the political body, and, in our case, there is the body body. That's what we are: miniature civic or provincial bodies, arguing every decision and action well into the night, fists pounding and voices hoarse. "No!" the blue, tight-lipped conservatives yell. "Yes!" the loose red liberals roar back. "Yes! Yes! Yes!"

In the body body, in most cases, it *is* the yes side that eventually wins. It's only a matter of time. If the smells and the urges can't put the bill through, they resort to the time-honoured political tool of propaganda. Among all of the other things going on in the unused real estate of the brain, somewhere back there, there is a history department that has no respect at all for what really happened.

When a child is eighteen months old, its parents are nervous wrecks. That child has tremendous speed, unrelenting curiosity and absolutely no sense of self-preservation. A lethal choking hazard is as much fun as a new doll, and so is an unguarded stairway. Naturally, that child's parents have difficulty fulfilling their individual potential and leading highly actualized lives. They are sleep-deprived, terrified, underfed, overweight zombies who haven't had a sensible conversation in well over a year and who can see nothing but potential calamity in any room they enter. They are ragged and grouchy and, doubtless, have sworn off the idea of having any more babies, no matter what else happens.

Then something else does happen: their kid grows up, and their brain erases all of those nasty memories. Once their toddler is out of diapers, parents miraculously decide that babies represent nothing but sweetness, purity and joy. All it takes is a neighbour's infant, or a stroller encounter, or (the most cruel) a nice dinner accompanied by a little adult conversation, and they are trapped again before you can say "to hell with social conformity."

And, if the internal propagandists can't erase the memory of toddler terror, other parents will.

"Oh, it was a wonderful time," older people are suddenly saying when they, for no reason, begin reminiscing about when they had their babies. It's just like that business of marriage being something "you have to work at." Talk about ruthless. They get all misty-eyed and smile those faraway smiles, not only disregarding the tyranny they are inflicting, but absolutely denying its existence. Jeff's plea "Go back, it's a trap" is far too kind. This is a conspiracy of lies, perpetrated by otherwise honest and respectable people in every corner of our society, and no one says a thing. The words "excruciating pain" or "pathological sleep loss" simply do not come up, and, especially, you will never hear a misty-eyed older person divulge parenthood's most basic and best-hidden truth: when you have a baby you automatically give away huge parts of yourself to a voracious and savage little tangle of cells, and those parts of yourself will never, ever be returned.

Ironically, that's also, in the end, what gets a parent through the ordeal. It's not what a baby takes, it's what he or she *will* take. The body body has one more trick to keep the system going when all others fail. It is the most powerful, the most relentless and the least understood of all. It is love.

Dr. George Bubenik, the endocrinologist at the University of Guelph who told me about the pheromones, also told me that very little is known about how much of parental love among humans is biological or neurological and how much is psychological. As a parent, it isn't hard to make a few educated guesses.

From the onset of puberty, most people are just dying to find someone who will accept their love. We learn through embarrassment and humiliation to keep our cards close to our chests with our fellow adults. We can show affection, even a little desire. But love is much bigger, and meaner, than that. It is voracious and savage, too. Those politicians who keep getting caught with their pants down will be tolerated for being driven to stupidity by their libidos. They may even admit to their dalliances and live to see another political day. But they will never admit to feeling love in any way except for the healthy, controlled kind that leads to speeches about their Lovely Wives and the Good Lord Above. For a human in a position of power to acknowledge true human love would be to admit weakness and subservience to a greater force. Love makes us into fools. We all know this. But, no matter how many deathbed proclamations we hear about the true nature of happiness, and how in the end each of us yearns only for love, nobody wants to admit it in front of anyone else.

With babies, all the rules go out the window. That's why the body body remembers early parenthood as such a wonderful time. It is such a relief to finally be able to pour out all of that love. Excruciating pain and sleep deprivation drift away into amnesia, while the feeling of finally being able to love without restriction never quite goes away. As a result, as with the best-thought-out traps, loving a child so much that it erases all other memory isn't actually unpleasant in the long run at all. And, if we end up liking it there, in the trap, and not wanting to leave, there is some philosophical question as to whether it is actually a trap at all.

That's what happened to my friend Jeff. As soon as his twin daughters were born, he naturally fell completely in love with them and forgot all his feelings of panic or regret. I called him that day I saw the couple necking on the park bench. The twins were just about to turn three, and he was more certain of his happiness than ever. In fact, he said, if such a thing is possible, he loved them even more than he had before.

Now, some might say that all of that love and emotion is simply part of the trap, that we are designed specifically to be inhibited with our love around other adults so that we will be all the more devoted to our babies' health and happiness, and therefore increase their chances of survival. It is possible that the highest expressions of emotion and spirituality and commitment, that the thousands of achingly beautiful melodies and paintings and poems fuelled by love, the very greatest creative achievements of the human race, are all just a part of one giant ruse from somewhere within the body body, perfectly designed to guarantee the continuation of the species.

I asked Jeff about that, if he ever wondered if all that love was just part of the trap, too, and he didn't hesitate. "Of course," he said. "But I don't care any more. I'm hooked."

The day after we talked, I saw the couple necking on the bench again. They came up for air at one point, and I had a good look at them. It was enchanting to see their faces. I got goosebumps just seeing the way they gazed into each other's eyes. I wanted to thank them. But I didn't. It was getting late, and I wanted to get home to see my kids.

Is That It?

I remember a cover story in *Modern Woman* magazine a few years ago. It was called "Men's Ten Biggest Fears." I don't remember very much about what was supposed to be so scary to me. The truth was, I was in a doctor's waiting room, and one of my biggest fears at the time was of getting caught reading *Modern Woman*. That one wasn't on the list. At least, I don't think it was. I flipped through the piece pretty quickly. I remember one fear was of going bald, which, for me, is like being afraid of waking up in the morning. Another was of finding that your penis is too small, which I'm not going to say anything about at all. Being afraid of writing about one's penis size wasn't on the list either. Call me chicken.

I became aware, though, at about fear number five ("I'll never be able to fix a flat as fast as my father"? "My wife is a better curler than me"? I wish I could remember . . .) that I'd been hoping for a kind of fun house thrill by reading this string of horrors, and it just wasn't happening. Even the fear about questioning sexuality ("I want to dress like a hydro worker"?) was laughable. I was about to throw the magazine down in disgust when I saw fear number ten. The boldface type leapt off the page. My stomach fell out the bottom of my pant leg. Three simple words, and I was a wreck.

"Is that it?"

That *was* it, as it turned out, for the article. That was all it needed. I have since read, I'm sure, works of great literature and journalism in publications of unquestionable merit, but those three words at the end of a mass-market one-pager have stayed with me ever since. Now and then they yell at me from the sidebars of my mind. "Is that it?" I wonder, when I am searching for a topic to write about and I come up with three or four that, my colleagues remind me, I have already used, sometimes twice. "Is that it?" I ask myself when I find that in my few quiet moments I have begun to reflect not on all of the many and wonderful things that still could happen in my life but on those that won't. Once you begin to think about it, "Is that it?" *is* it. It won't leave you alone.

Clearly, these days, there *are* more concrete things to be worried about, regardless of your gender. What used to be the middle class has become the working poor, and what was once a troubled home has become just another cover story for the local tabloids. Hospitals close and shelters fill, bankruptcies soar, crime follows, and downsizing claims victim after victim, who, in most cases, were just getting going when they found they were gone.

Even less comforting is the one-stop solution an increasing number of people seem to be choosing: buy a minivan with an alarm system, live in a gated community and never leave your vehicle until you have arrived in the secure, underground parking lot of your downtown office.

But the one thing the minivan, the alarm system, the automatic garage-door-opener, the 4,000-square-foot house with the cathedral ceiling on the cul-de-sac with the rent-a-cops parked at every bend cannot protect me, or anyone else, from is insignificance, and that, safe to say, is scary for most of us.

As for myself, I know exactly where my fear of insignificance comes from. I've been raised with, or have genetically inherited, a self-worth that is directly processed through the culture of adventure.

I don't think I am alone in this. Movies and television are full of programs that play on our basic need to see ourselves as adventurers. There is an entire genre of film based on the idea that an average person can go from an everyday life situation to suddenly being in the midst of life-threatening danger. Soap operas have stayed on the air for decades by portraying ordinary human relationships as wild, unpredictable vehicles for fantastic swings between the highest good and the deepest evil. There is even a game show that turns the mundane chore of checking prices in the grocery store into an opportunity for fabulous winnings! If the entertainment industry is any indication of our appetite for the culture of adventure, we are ripe for the picking.

This is not an easy thing for me to point out. Almost all of my most dearly treasured memories and achievements hang on the belief in my own life's adventure. I loved walking through Central Park when I lived in New York. It was the beginning of my adult life. I was working. I was living on my own. Here was this famous place I'd seen in movies so many times, the great, thronging centre of the continent's most powerful city. New York City! Buildings! History! Charm and elegance and money and power, and there I was, right in the middle of it—a man on his own, an adventurer in the great voyage of life.

Years later, after I'd moved back to Canada and married, my wife and I visited New York for a weekend holiday. Here was my chance to show my worldliness, for her to see what a catch she had made by netting the adventurous and sophisticated former New Yorker. We went to Central Park and walked slowly across, taking in its every greatness.

"But," she said, after a while, "it's dirty."

"It's Central Park!" I offered.

"It's old."

"It's . . ." I offered, again, "Central Park!"

"I'm hungry," she said. "Is that it?"

Is that it? Evidently, if it's not your adventure, that's it.

An awful truth dawned on me that day in the waiting room reading *Modern Woman*: maybe the delusion of adventure is the only thing that makes *anything* more than "it." Maybe, I wondered, we manufacture this sense of adventure to bring on the delusion of significance, without which we would simply cease to function. It is a horrible thought. If we are only adventuring to pad our slim self-image, then what we are pursuing is, in fact, merely the *perception* of adventure. If that is so, then there is no longer any difference between hiking across the African savanna and going to Busch Gardens, or between climbing Mount Fuji and taking the escalator to the food court for a Teriyaki Wrap at Samurai Sammy's.

The one factor, as far as I can figure, that separates the perception of adventure from actual adventure is risk.

Hiking across the African savanna is still actually dangerous. Busch Gardens, beyond the threat of millions of unfortunately clothed and deluded adventurers breathing through their mouths, is not. In the savanna there are carnivorous beasts who are in no way deluded as to their own significance, or yours. They are starving, and you are dinner. As for climbing Mount Fuji, it might not be as fraught with mystery and danger for North Americans as it once was, but there are still things happening there that you won't find back in the food court.

So, if real danger is what defines adventure and therefore saves us from self-deception and insignificance, the good news is that we don't have to go anywhere to find it any more—it is coming after us! Choking pollutants poison the atmosphere! Cancerous ooze boils from the ground! Nature reels with hypothermic ice storms and freakish summer snows! Flesh-eating bacteria laugh off flaccid antibiotics! And, in the city, packs of angry youths armed like terrorists lurk along boarded-up streets, while trigger-happy SWAT teams descend from the rooftops, flaying law-abiding citizens for crosswalk violations and overly noisy lawnmowers. There are so many things to be afraid of now, it's positively terrifying.

But what is *really* scary to me is not all of that danger. It's that it isn't any fun any more.

I can remember going to see *Apocalypse Now* just after my eighteenth birthday. The sign said I had to be that old to get in. Others might have celebrated legal age with a drinking binge, or by revelling in their newly acquired power as a voter, or both. Not me. I was a free-thinking adult, paying good money to be scared out of my wits. And not just there's-a-bad-guy-behind-the-door-with-a-cleaver scared. No. I wanted real, the-world-is-a-horrible-twisted-place-and-there-are-no-easy-answers scared. I wanted discomfort. I wanted anxiety. I got them. It was great.

For youth, danger and fear and anxiety and discomfort are the best things going. They are proof that life is finally real. Young people are so good with anxiety that each generation searches and searches until it finds a new strain that will bring them great excitement and simultaneously terrify, and distance, their parents. These days it is body-piercing and tattoos; a couple of decades ago it was wild hair and toxic stimulants; before that it was impossibly fast cars and games of "chicken" on the public roads. And, throughout, youth writes the soundtrack. There is nothing to spur on the youthful quest for danger like whatever mind-bending, ear-splitting music has been chosen as the noise *du jour*.

I never thought I would tire of Led Zeppelin, and John Bonham's[1] deadly drumming still does give me a real thrill, but the lyrics, even with Robert Plant's searing range, somehow, fail to reflect much of my outlook on life now. It might be because of one too many lines about big-legged women, or perhaps I am tired of wondering just how alarmed I should be if there's a bustle in my hedgerow. I don't know.

Nevertheless, after straying from Led Zeppelin, my ears used some kind of natural selection process until the only stuff left from my salad days were the wilted greens.

---

[1] He was truly a genius, and he has even been recognized as such in the crusty halls of academe. My friend Dave Gier was doing his Doctor of Musical Arts degree at Yale when he noted "Led Zeppelin was a rhythmically stable ensemble." His adviser nodded gravely.

And the scary part is, I still like them. James Taylor has, to me, one of the most naturally beautiful and expressive voices in popular music. But I know, even as I listen to him singing and am filled with comfort and happiness, that to anyone more than five years younger than I am, I might as well be hearing Doris (I'm sorry to say this, James) Day. In fact, those younger people would actually *rather* hear Doris Day. The crooners that made my eyes roll around more than a mirror-ball at a high school dance are now considered retro-hip.

Granted, even back in my thorny youth, James Taylor's music was probably not what I would have chosen to bring on great pains and anxiety and an overwhelming urge to go out and do something life-threatening. But that is the point. Without warning me, my own subconscious has wilfully deleted any vitality from my repertoire, to the point that the only music left from my youth is designed not to bring on anxiety but to diffuse it.

Movies are the same. I found that out watching *Alive*. It wasn't about the futility of human life. It wasn't an endless boat trip into the swamp of human cruelty and the madness of war. It was about a soccer team whose plane crashes in the Andes and how several of them manage to survive. Okay, they have to eat a few of the dead to do so. At least it had a happy ending. No matter. In the fourteen years since I had seen *Apocalypse Now*, and, more to the point, in the three months since I had become a father, I'd become a suck. Seeing *Alive* shook me badly. I left the theatre feeling like I'd barely survived a plane crash myself, and, to my great shock, I had to admit that I didn't like it.

For a former adventurer, this was bad news. I was in no position to be losing my significance. I was a father! And if the culture of adventure ruled that discomfort/anxiety/fear/danger was what I needed to keep that significance, I wasn't sure how much more I could take.

Discomfort—I was miserable! I hadn't slept more than three hours in weeks, and when I did, between the baby and the pillows and the blankets, I'd wake up clinging to the edge of the bed as if I were ready to fall off the Andes myself.

Anxiety—I was a wreck! The first time the baby slept through the night I was up fifteen times to make sure he was still alive.

Fear—I was terrified! There were so many things waiting to go wrong it was stupefying! What if my son inherited my forgetfulness, my irresponsibility or my bad jump shot?

Danger—well, that was the rub. The danger, and whatever adventurous significance it carried with it, was no longer mine. Our baby might have made me uncomfortable, anxious and fearful, but he wasn't going to kill me. In fact, I couldn't see any danger for myself at all, any more. But for him, it was everywhere. I'd never known how dangerous the world was. Forget about cancerous ooze—what about sudden bursts of cold air? What about faulty car seats and high chairs? Or little tiny bits of teriyaki stuff that could choke a baby while his unwary parent tried to relax for a moment in the food court?

I guess that's when danger stopped being fun. Suddenly, danger wasn't the exception any more, it ruled.

That was six years ago. Since then, of course, as every other parental generation has, I have been caught in the conundrum of the culture of adventure. I want my children to embrace life, to learn to grab hold of whatever comes their way, and in my heart, I know I would be proud if they eventually did choose to hike across the African savanna—but I can't bear the thought of the danger. On the other hand, if they go to Busch Gardens, or whatever disgusting equivalent is pressed upon the hapless boobs of tomorrow, as a former adventurer turned parent, I can only count myself as a failure.

And when they do go wherever they are going, what will be left for me? By then, I will have been so incapacitated by vicarious adventuring and terrifying, ubiquitous danger that, I'm sure, my own taste for discomfort/fear/anxiety/danger will be as tiny as a tortilla on Mount Fuji. I will want a nice, big bed every night, no matter where I am. I will want an alarm system on my cathedral-ceilinged monster home. I will want a minivan to take me away from the boarded-up streets of the city. I will want my tax break at the expense of hospital beds for the mentally ill. I will call adventurous young people communists/hippies/squeegee kids, or whatever stupid term the geezer-boomers will come up with, and I will defend my consuming appetite for saccharine melodies and harmless, chirpy movies by saying, "I don't know much about music (or movies, ballet, art, architecture, theatre, tattoos or body piercing), but I know what I like."

The horror.

But that, according to the culture of adventure, is also the good news.

Because if fear is what makes a real adventure real, and if real adventure is the criteria for significance, then, logically, the prospect of insignificance, if it causes enough fear, results in real adventure and, ultimately, significance.

So, is that it?

Well, I don't know, but I'm willing to look into it. It's not that I want any of those unpleasant things in my life, particularly, but if fear/danger/discomfort/anxiety is what makes me significant, I'm doing pretty well already. And, the way I look at it, if I start feeling too complacent, I can always go to the doctor's office and pick up a copy of *Modern Woman*.

Dearly Departed

As a distinguished author nearing the end of his first book, I would like to be able to address the topic of death with something other than screaming, white-knuckle terror. But I would be lying, about dying, if I did. I am not ready to die. I am not even ready to understand why I am not ready. If I do die before I'm ready, as that far-too-cool-in-the-face-of-death young man played by Leonardo DiCaprio in *Titanic* pointed out, there will be a strongly worded letter in the mail the very next day.

My dad has a joke that I've appropriated more and more of late. A man wakes up on a Monday morning and, glancing through the newspaper, he is surprised to find an obituary in his own name. As he reads on, his astonishment increases. The person listed as having died over the weekend not only had his name but was his precise age, shared many of his interests and is survived by the same number and gender of children. The man decides he'd better call some of his friends, in case they have read the obit too.

"Frank?" he says to his buddy at the office. "It's Bob, I thought I'd better call you after that obituary appeared in the paper."

"Yeah." Frank says. "I read it. Where are you calling from?"

And how much did the call cost? Furthermore, what if the deceased wasn't calling just to say "Hi," but to let his friend know things weren't quite what he'd hoped: that the cabins are small and the service is slow and there seems to be an awful lot of water coming up from steerage? *Will* the afterlife be the kind of place to tolerate letters of complaint to the management? If not, I have to wonder what kind of Paradise it could possibly be.

I also wonder, once I get there, if I'll be able to find my cat.

Scooter died in the summer of 1996. He was twelve and a half years old, and still King of the Hill. The last time I saw him he was chasing some black-and-white punk off our front walk. His kidneys failed three days later.

I still miss him.

I miss the way he'd bump into my leg while I did the dishes. I miss the way he'd plow his paws into the quilt in the middle of the night and raise the temperature under the covers to about 400 degrees Celsius. And yes, I guess I miss him waking me up in the middle of the night so he could tear out and clobber every other feline on the street.

Scooter was my wife's cat, first. By the time I showed up he'd lived in nine different places. That number reached sixteen before he died. Maybe that's why he was such a scrapper. He'd had to work his way to the top more times than Sir Edmund Hillary.

In Halifax we lived in an upstairs flat. Scooter had to jump eight feet to get to our balcony door. He thought about it for months before he tried. In fact, I think the day he finally did it was after we'd hired him out as a mercenary. The downstairs neighbours, our landlords, had mice. They weren't cat people. They just wanted the job done, and they were prepared to pay: tuna, right from the can. Scooter bagged three in half an hour. Later that night he jumped the eight feet up to the balcony. All in a day's work.

It's in Halifax that I remember him most. We didn't know anybody. We didn't have kids yet. We were lonely. "He's just a cat," I'd tell myself when I called him to come in at night. We lived on a busy street. I'd seen him run across the road without looking first. He did it all the time. So, I'd stand up there in the doorway, whistling and calling and waking up the neighbours, with the pit in my stomach getting harder by the second, wondering if he'd finally done himself in and we'd lost him for good.

And then he'd nip up that eight-foot jump, cruise in the door and ask for a snack.

I still look for him now and then. When I run the can opener, I half expect to hear him bellowing at me as he pounds down the stairs. And I think of him when my kids ask me where he went.

I've said he's in Cat Heaven, of course, which I certainly would like to think is true, but, when pressed to offer details of his life there, the logic of the idea begins to break down. If I think of what appeared to be pleasurable to him in this life, Scooter's Heaven would undoubtedly include someone to open the door at all hours of the night, food provided on demand, very quiet children, if any, and lots of slow-running mice and near-sighted dogs.

At first, this all seems possible using a sort of apocalyptic food-chain model, in which Scooter's Heaven might also simultaneously function as a kind of Dog and Mouse

Hell. The condemned dogs are given poor sight and no sense of smell, so that they can see well enough to give chase and provide the virtuous cats with much entertainment and exercise, but pose no actual danger. The mice are much the same, except, instead of being quarrors, they are quarry, and because of their lack of speed they are soon quarnered and quartered.

But the numbers won't add up. The mice condemned to Mouse Hell/Cat Heaven, naturally, would be eaten at a tremendous rate, causing supply problems. Surely there could be no shortage of mice in Cat Heaven. But if, on the other hand, the mice are to be recycled in Mouse Hell—that is, perpetually killed and reborn only to be consumed again (as is often the case in Hell-like scenarios—and must be so, or their time in Hell would be so short as to be less Hellish than life on Earth)—there would be far too many bad mice for even a very good cat like Scooter to catch and consume, making things considerably less than Heavenly for the poor, hard-working and virtuous cat.

There is also the question of whether there is such a thing as a good cat, or bad mouse, at all. To a cat owner, a good cat is one that is ruthless and savage and takes great delight in the murder of other beings that have committed no crime other than being where they are on the food chain. Even mice, although I am not at all keen on having them in my house, are not inherently evil. They are probably, in the grand and natural scheme of things, much less so than I. They are not plotting my demise with ruthless and savage carnivorous pets that would take great delight in slowly killing me and chewing me up, leaving only shards of my bones in a pile near the front door beside little bits of what was once my head. At least, I don't think they are. Nor are they, as far as I know, setting my daily routes with giant mechanical traps, baited with irresistible treats and equipped with great, swooping wire bars designed specifically to crush my spine instantly. A mouse of such dark character would deserve to be condemned to an afterlife as a permanent afternoon snack. No. Mice are just mice. They are hungry, and when they get cold they come into your house. That's all.

Is it impossible, then, that a similar standard could exist for humans? Despite our capacity for guilt and what passes for reason—or at least rationalization, perhaps—in our earthly lives, we are simply putting into action some standard-issue human characteristics: cruelty, selfishness, destruction and irresponsibility, and a deep capacity for evil. That's just the way it is.

Unfortunately, or perhaps fortunately, in most visions of an afterlife, enlightenment, saintliness, moral integrity or, at the very least, some sort of last-minute admission of something less than perfection are non-negotiable prerequisites. In fact, as impossible as it might seem to transcend human behaviour while one is, after all, only human, the idea of some kind of judgment against that very behaviour is necessary to the belief in any kind of afterlife at all. Otherwise, it could easily be no different than the duringlife, and all the cheaters and hosers and liars and people who act like, well, human beings, instead of mice, would be up there in Heaven too, and it wouldn't be Heaven at all.

At times I envision a web-like condominium society, in which there are many floors and levels (some with sunken conversation pits with gas fireplaces) and adjoining passageways that sort and separate the various levels of former humanity into workable communities. Because, aside from our intrinsic amorality as humans, I do believe we can be sorted into levels of Heavenliness. I can think of a number of people who, after even a few minutes together, leave me feeling buoyant and confident, with a full heart and, you might say, even spiritually refreshed. They seem to be able to do this at no cost to themselves, and often it appears that they, too, are recharged by the very experience of recharging.

There are also those who are precisely the opposite, people who drain the soul within a few seconds of small talk, as if, whatever energy of the soul or heart this is I am trying to identify, they are in a constant state of deficit. I don't like being with people like that. I will walk a long way to avoid them. But that is not to say I think they deserve to be damned to burn eternally in Hell, or even in the paridisal gas fireplace. I just don't want to end up stuck beside them in the conversation pit. Not even for a moment, let alone until the end of time.

So, what about the notion of a multi-level community? I'm assuming that the tiny number of truly virtuous souls holding the club record for transcendent human virtue at one end of the human goodness continuum, and Adolf Hitler and all of his thousands of neighbours at the other end, will have communities all their own, with appropriate admission standards and activities.[1] But for the rest of us, being a child of the '70s, I envision some sort of vertical dwelling. If it hadn't been used so many times already, I'd call it "Heaven's most exclusive location," or "prestigious downtown living" or something like that.

---

[1] I'll admit I'm glossing over a rather large philosophical point, here. There is still the enormous question of how close to either Hitler or

The vast majority of souls—those of us who muddled along through life, occasionally helping others and about as often hurting—would all live in the huge mid-layer, say, on floors three to fifty. The few and precious soul-rechargers might live together in wonderful pools of light on the airy and brilliant fifty-first floor, but they could still wander down to the mid-level areas now and then to do the wonderful recharging they so enjoy. And the blood-sucking, parasitical and snivelling, although not completely evil, soul-drainers would stay down in the basement to deal, since they're so good at it, with the occasional drainage problem, but now and then they would still stumble on minimal access to the general population and be invited to the annual picnic, at the last minute, with the hope that they will have already made other plans.

I wouldn't want to be the superintendent of such a dwelling, I'll admit. But, according to most religious ideologies, that job is already taken, anyway. Let's hope St. Peter, if that's who it is, has a head for business. And an up-to-date phone list. Just like the guy in my father's joke, there are a few people I'll be wanting to get hold of soon after I check in.

There's Doug Shanks. Doug was a retired United Church minister when I met him. He sang only one cowboy song on my phone machine before he died. It was "When the Work's All Done this Fall." He accompanied himself on the autoharp. I'd like to hear more.

---

the ideal human one would have to be on the good/evil continuum before any permanent placement were made, and where to put those that are just on the inside of those points of decision. But I'm trying to move things along. If I'm wrong about this, I'll let you know when I get there. If I'm allowed to use the phone.

My grandmother was a lifelong member of the Plymouth Brethren, a fundamentalist sect that frowns on dancing and any music that isn't directed toward the glorification of the Almighty. She shocked me one day when I heard her humming along with me from the kitchen as I picked out Duke Ellington's "Sophisticated Lady" on the piano. I wonder what other tunes she knows.

Millie Hubbert told me about her first Christmas fruitcake. She found the recipe, got about halfway through and, when she came back from finding some ingredient from the back of her fridge, failed to notice that in her absence a breeze had flipped over a few pages of her cookbook. She ended up with something that was one half "Classic Christmas Treat" and the other "Company Rumcake Surprise." She said it was pretty good, but I never got to try it. I'd like to. Mostly, though, I'd like to hear her tell me the story again.

I am also determined to see, once again, someone who, I am certain, lives in the brightest and airiest of all the rooms on the fifty-first floor.

I have Josh's picture on the wall above my desk. He's sitting cross-legged on the floor, with a faraway smile and a French horn in his lap. Josh died of a rare form of cancer in 1991. He was nineteen. I still catch myself talking about him as if he were alive.

I'm also still angry about losing him. Because, although I'm still working out where to put everybody, and I joke about how ridiculous the idea of any kind of Heaven is, when humans are involved, I do believe some kind of higher order is at play in this world. It is difficult to justify at times, I'll admit. Most of the time, in fact. I can't imagine any good reason for Josh's dying. It turns any argument, logical or otherwise, for the belief in any kind of all-powerful, or even somewhat conscious, God into hollow and patronizing platitudes. Josh's death was wrong in every way. It was criminal and stupid and awful and makes absolutely no sense to me at all.

But even with his family and friends, who have surely suffered far more grief than I have or ever will, every time we talk about Josh, we laugh.

Josh was a big, wonderful, goofy guy. He had wisdom far beyond his years and a heart the size of a kettledrum. Love just fell out of him. All he had to do was look at you. And he lived with music in a way I've never seen before or since. He never had any training. He just understood it. And not only the music other nineteen-year-olds were listening to at the time—although he liked that fine, too. His real passion was for the excessive and blasting romantics: Bruckner, Mahler, Sibelius and Brahms. Most people, if they're ever going to learn to love that stuff, don't do it until they are well into their forties, when all that honking is a faint reminder of delicious former passions, the kind they enjoyed when they were nineteen. Josh didn't need to wait to know how to hear all that passion, which, considering his early death, seems a little too coincidental.

The French horn he's holding in the picture on my wall was a piece of junk. A friend gave it to him. It was old and tarnished and dented, and getting any sound out of it was like blowing on your thumb. But one afternoon, on my way to a rehearsal at the church we sang in, I happened upon Josh, alone in the sanctuary, in the dark, making so much noise on that busted up old horn you could hear him halfway down the block. He'd only tried to play it for the first time that afternoon, and it didn't sound too bad.

Then he showed it to me, and I found the valves were seized shut with rust.

A few months later he told me he was playing that same horn in a student musical—second horn in a theatre orchestra. He had the valves working by then, but he still couldn't read music. He just figured it out.

That was at King's College in Halifax. Josh started his BA there. So, when we moved there too, at the start of his second year, I couldn't wait to see him. But it was September, and all the students were arriving at once. I didn't know his address. There was a waiting list to get a phone installed and I didn't know how to tell him where I was living. Then one night, two or three days after we'd moved in, I came home after work and there was a cheque lying on the floor in the entrance room, dropped through the mail slot. I still have it. It's made out in my name, for the sum of one cent, written numerically, too: $00.01. It's signed Joshua Julian Barnes, and, on the little memo line in the lower left-hand corner, there is a note: "Re: thoughts."

No phone number, no address, just a penny for my thoughts.

He turned up for dinner the next night.

Food comes up in a lot of my memories, almost as much as music—he *was* nineteen, after all. We once sat in the cold on a park bench in Halifax, on a damp November night, long after midnight, eating donairs. We'd just finished listening to all of Mahler's Seventh Symphony in Josh's dorm room at ear-splitting volume. It was the great Chicago Symphony/Sir Georg Solti recording from the early '70s, the one with Adolph "Bud" Herseth rising out of the pack of trumpets in the final movement like Buck

Rogers, Maynard Ferguson, Robin Hood and Sheriff Matt Dillon all rolled into one. We'd been competing with some head-bangers listening to something dinosaur-like in the room below, but they gave up after Herseth's high C in the fourth time through the theme in the Rondo. Then we went for donairs.

Donairs are a Halifax junk food specialty. They're made of a chewy meat-like substance that is singed all day on a vertical electric spit. The donair-*donneurs* slice off the flesh in hunks and drop the whole greasy mess into foil-wrapped pita bread, liberally glopped with toxic garlic sauce. The only acceptable posture for eating a donair is hunched forward with your knees far enough apart to escape the inevitable slop that cascades from your chin. Even then your hands smell like the sidewalk on garbage day for the next two weeks. It took me ten minutes to convince Josh to try his. Then he went back and bought us seconds.

"Some friend," he said later. "That stuff probably gave me cancer."

His funeral was hard. I sang in the choir. I thought it would help because I'd be doing something for him, at least. He loved music so much. But my voice wouldn't work. I opened my mouth and nothing came out at all.

A few weeks later, though, there was a memorial service at King's College, in the chapel. King's is a pretty stiff old place—all those Anglican rituals. Josh used to say they couldn't afford a football team because they spent all the money on the Bishop's yearly supply of bejewelled bangles and exotic gold vestments.

But even King's relaxed a bit for Josh in that service. One of his friends improvised a nonsense song with a margarine tub for accompaniment. There was a reading about beets—Josh's favourite vegetable. The passage was from the Tom Robbins book *Jitterbug Perfume*, and it ends with the memorable claim that "Only the beet departs your body the same color as when it went in."[2] And Josh's roommate played a blues number on the harmonica. "Don't worry 'bout me," the old song goes, "I'm sittin' on top of the world."

I have no doubt.

When I step back a little bit, this all seems like a flimsy foundation on which to build a faith—to swallow the urge to wonder, if there is an all-powerful being worth anything close to His heavenly weight, how He can sleep at night. Maybe He's beyond sleep now, or maybe He doesn't have time to fit it in. Maybe He's too busy trying to save brilliant and gifted and almost-too-wonderful-for-this-world nineteen-year-olds with cancer. I don't know. But I'll forgive God for that, and the rest, if I can be allowed the faint and wonderful hope that I'll one day get to hear Mahler blasted out of a college dorm in the middle of the night and go out for donairs again. I know, just like the mice, on a moral scale, it probably doesn't add up. I don't care. I'm willing to take that chance.

But sometimes I get tired of waiting for him to call.

Then again, there probably won't be too many others up there on the fifty-first, I don't think. Not in my Heaven, anyway. And even if there are, I'll just listen for

---

[2] The passage concludes: "The lesson of the beet, then, is this: Hold onto your divine blush, your innate rosy magic, or end up brown. Once you're brown, you'll find that you're blue. As blue as indigo. And you know what that means: Indigo. Indigoing. Indigone."

the blasting Mahler's Third Symphony, or maybe the French horn. My guess is, whatever few earthly limitations Josh was burdened with in his short life, he isn't worrying about them now. He can probably already sight-read like a demon[3], and play anything he wants to, at any hour of the day or night.

Some of the folks down below might get tired of it, I suppose, just like they did back here all those years ago. But, seeing as it's Heaven where they are, it probably wouldn't be worth complaining about. Who complains in Heaven? Besides, the noise probably keeps away the mice.

---

[3] You wouldn't think anyone would be doing anything like a demon in Heaven, but that's the expression among musicians as I've heard it: "Reads like a demon." There's also "Sings like an angel," "Plays like a god," and, in jazz, "Blows like the devil." Maybe there's lots of time to practise in Heaven, and sight-reading isn't necessary. Maybe all the jazz clubs are in the basement.

A Short Footnote[1] on Footnotes

As you will have noticed by now, unless you have started reading on this page,[2] I have written this book with the use of footnotes. I'll be honest, I'm only using them because my word processor[3] has a "footnote" feature, which is kind of cool, and because I like the way Paul Quarrington used them[4] in his latest book.[5]

But as I was writing, at least for the first few pages, to continue being honest,[6] I felt a little guilty about the whole thing. In the past, I thought that the only legitimate footnote was one that was used to provide more information about the source of a given literary quote or reference[7] than space and readability would allow within the main body of the text. Any other use of footnotes, to

---

[1] See?

[2] And if you brushed past this piece's title, and first line, and began reading on the word "page."

[3] WordPerfect 6.0, purchased on sale, including a nifty graphics package, for $48 at Business Depot, on University Avenue in Toronto.

[4] To very humorous effect.

[5] *The Boy On the Back of the Turtle* (Toronto: GreyStone Books, 1997).

[6] Why stop now?

[7] Like the one before last.

me, was self-indulgence. If the material was worth including at all, I reasoned, it was worth including it along with everything else. Otherwise, it simply looked pretentious.[8]

But I was wrong.[9] I've just looked up "footnote"[10] in the *Concise Oxford English Dictionary*,[11] and it says that a footnote is a "note inserted at foot of page." That's all. Isn't that great?[12] Footnotes aren't an exclusively academic tool after all. They have nothing to do with credibility,[13] only the geography of the page. I've got a mind to use them even more often[14] from now on.

The trouble is, in this book,[15] I've been finding it's very easy to let the footnotes get out of control.[16] They're so easy to use.[17] And there is humour[18] in having[19] the narrative move from up[20] to down and back,[21] at the author's

---

[8] He's telling us?

[9] I know we're just the plebes down here, but that does strike this footnote as a good reason for not bringing it up in the first place.

[10] Page 381, before "Footpace" (walking pace) and after "Footmuff" (for keeping foot warm).

[11] Oxford University Press, 1982 edition, reprinted 1984.

[12] Oh boy.

[13] As if there was any doubt about that by now.

[14] You'll notice he never worried about the credibility of all those words "up there."

[15] *Toe Rubber Blues* by Tom Allen (Toronto: Penguin Books, 1999).

[16] And that's *our* fault?

[17] So were indentured servants.

[18] And who says *he* gets to decide when we get to say anything, anyway?

[19] Or how big our font is?!

[20] Narrative, shmarrative! The whole idea of "footnotes" and "main text" is prejudicial to begin with. Why is it considered intrinsically inferior to be at the bottom of the page, anyway?

[21] And *is* it a given that a person wouldn't read the footnote first? What about from down to up and back again? This is one of those North/South things Trudeau was always talking about.

will, regardless of payoff.[22] But, in the final diagnosis,[23] [24] [25] it is this writer's opinion[26] that footnotes[27] can be used[28] with a clear conscience,[29] and a full heart,[30] and[31] a[32] modicum[33] of[34] restraint.[35]

[22] Payoff? Ha!

[23] Arthur Hailey (New York: Doubleday, 1959).

[24] Oops. Damn. That was a regression. He'll never take me seriously now.

[25] Maybe I could find work in a university press somewhere.

[26] Nothing too fancy. Somewhere with margins. Maybe the Midwest.

[27] It just might be nice to be treated with a little respect.

[28] My dad was in medicine, with the *New England Journal.*

[29] He died in a report on myocardial infarction.

[30] It was the syllables.

[31] So, I don't know. Academia might be too stressful.

[32] I could check out the government publishers.

[33] It could even be a report on hospital closings, or something. I don't care if anyone ever reads it.

[34] It's just that, after all the talking's done, I wouldn't mind if there were something left for me, something to hold on to.

[35] Because, in the end, even if it's only in ten-point Janson Roman, and below the text line at the very bottom of the last page of the epilogue, I guess I'm not really looking for all that much. It's just nice to have a chance, once in a while, to get in the last word.